THE
HEALING
JOURNEY

THROUGH MENOPAUSE

Your Journal for
Reflection and Renewal

Phil Rich, EdD, MSW
Fran Mervyn, BSN, PhD

John Wiley & Sons, Inc.

NEW YORK ✦ CHICHESTER ✦ WEINHEIM ✦ BRISBANE ✦ SINGAPORE ✦ TORONTO

ISBN 0-471-32691-7

Printed in the United States of America.

10 9 8 7 6 5 4 3 2 1

Contents

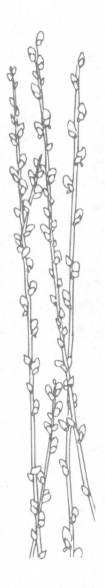

PREFACE

About *The Healing Journey Through Menopause*

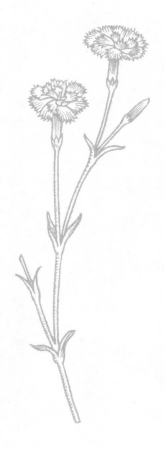

UNTIL RECENTLY IN our culture, passage through menopause was a silent and solitary experience. This change of life was often perceived negatively, especially in those times and places where a woman's worth was tied to her reproductive capacity. In the first part of this century, menopausal women with mood shifts or depressive symptoms were diagnosed with "involutional melancholia," and some were even committed to mental institutions. Menopause was associated with sickness, aging, and loss of sexuality. No wonder it was greeted with fear and denial.

For millions of women who were introduced to their menstrual cycle as "the curse," menopause was another curse, but more silent. Today women are working on transcending these negative perceptions.

Masses of baby boomers are now entering their forties and fifties. Despite the general daily risk to health we all face, some statistics tell us that a healthy fifty-year-old woman today has a life expectancy of ninety-two. With these changes in both population and improved health, the perception and experience of menopause is also changing. Where there once was little or no information, interest, or intervention, there are now numerous sources for both research and theory. Where there were once only negative phrases associated with menopause, such as "wizened" and "dried up," there are now alternate and more optimistic ways to describe the experience. The nationally syndicated columnist Ellen Goodman coined the phrase *menopositive,* and hot flashes are now often referred to as "power surges." Perimenopause (premenopause) is the "springtime of the rest of your life," according to Dr. Christiane Northrup, a well-known health educator and medical practitioner. Asked how she could be so energetic in her fifties and sixties, Dr. Margaret Mead answered, "Post-menopausal zest!"

So what does all this mean for you? It means that the more you take this real opportunity to know the person you used to be (physically, mentally, and emotionally), the more you will discover your inner resources and the more rich will your experience be of the person you are becoming. You can use to your advantage the "pause" as an invitation to stop and take stock of your life and health before launching into the years ahead. Even if your signs of menopause are few, the opportunity for reflection that this life stage may offer you can be beneficial for long-term health and well-being.

Most likely you're experiencing some physical changes about which you have questions. You wonder about menopause and what it will mean for you. *The Healing Journey Through Menopause* is a guided personal journal that will help you understand and work through the process in a way that's best for you. Whether your experience of menopause is a breeze or a storm, the experience of working through what it means to you will stand you in good stead for the rest of your life. Understanding this change in your body and this time in your life will help you make informed decisions about who you are and who you want to become. This journal can be your confidant, a guidebook that is just for you as you move forward in your life.

I

Embarking on Your Journey

DURING THIS DECADE, menopause has become a major topic of discussion. This shift from silent to strong voice has been shaped by many forces, but among the most influential is the sheer number of women now encountering menopause. If you're in your forties or fifties, you're among this baby-boom generation, the largest group ever to enter menopause in the United States.

Menopause can be a defining life experience, a springboard to the second half of your life. If you're one of the millions of women now anticipating or encountering the changes that accompany this stage of human development, *The Healing Journey Through Menopause* will assist you in charting your own passage in your own way.

Whether you're just entering this life passage (perimenopause), have been catapulted into it through a medical procedure (such as radiation or removal of the ovaries), or have ceased menstruating for a whole year now (officially then, menopause), this book can assist you in coming to terms with where you are and what you need to think about to make this phase of your life, which could last a decade or more, an opportunity for renaissance and re-

"Women over fifty already form one of the largest groups in the population structure of the western world. As long as they like themselves, they will not be an oppressed minority. In order to like themselves they must reject trivialization by others of who and what they are. A grown woman should not have to masquerade as a girl in order to remain in the land of the living."
— GERMAINE GREER

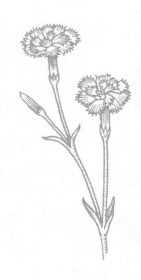

newal. Even if you're past menopause and have acclimated to the physical changes it brought, you'll find this book helpful in reflecting on what this adjustment has meant to your life.

Planning Your Journey

How do you make sense of all that's available along your own journey? First, you have to be discerning. Most people simply can't consume all the material that's out there, so they have to be selective in the first place just to figure out what to read and to whom to listen. But if you have the energy, time, and interest, read what's available, check out Internet sites, watch talk shows, and listen to experts on the subject. The more informed you are, the better able you'll be to make the kind of choices that make the most sense for you. Choose the ideas and suggestions that seem to best answer your questions and fit your needs. Find a health care practitioner whose approach and values most closely match your own and in whose opinions you trust.

The more informed you are, the better able you'll be to make the kind of choices that make the most sense for you.

Second, become aware of your physical, emotional, intellectual, and spiritual needs. Without self-awareness it is difficult to be discerning. As you read, listen, and generally sort through all these menopause resources, *interact* with what you're learning. Consider the relevance of specific material to your life and your needs. Think about what you're learning about *yourself* as you absorb all this new information.

The Healing Journey Through Menopause will help you explore your needs, experiment with your ideas, and figure out how you want to approach this change in your life. It will provide you with a means for looking at your own experience and discovering your inner coping style, attitudes, and preferences. Understanding your own needs can help you not only make better use of all those available resources but also help you pick materials, products, and ideas that most fit your own ideas.

Keeping a Journal

A journal can meet many needs. In its most basic form, a journal is a way to record the details of your life; it is a memoir of your experiences and thoughts. A journal can also be a special companion —a part of yourself that exists outside of you in which you share your feelings, your ideas, your worries, and your successes. Beyond this, a journal can be a place to explore and express your thoughts and feelings, reflect on the way you interact with the people and things that surround you, and experiment with new ideas. Journal writing becomes a means to record and better understand how you approach life and how you *want* to approach life.

A *guided* journal, like *The Healing Journey Through Menopause*, goes one step further. Interspersed with relevant ideas and information, it introduces you to journaling and provides structured journal entries that will help you discover and express your feelings, frame your thoughts, and experiment with different journaling styles and techniques. Ultimately, a journal can be a valuable companion along a deeply personal road.

Much of the benefit of *The Healing Journey Through Menopause* comes from gaining skills in reflection and self-expression. As you answer questions or write your thoughts in a journal entry, you're having a "conversation" with yourself. Even if you have a problem expressing your thoughts and feelings to others, writing can be cathartic, allowing you to unburden yourself in private. The main thing is that you *are* expressing what you think and feel.

Your journal can be of great value as you work through the issues surrounding menopause. It can help you understand what you need at whatever stage in the process you find yourself. Using it on a regular basis will enhance your ability to make this change your own, proceeding at your own pace and learning what is important for *you*.

Journal writing becomes a means to record and better understand how you approach life and how you want to approach life.

Moving Through *The Healing Journey Through Menopause*

Although menopause signals the end of one life phase and the beginning of another, that change doesn't take place overnight.

If you're working with a counselor or other health care professional, she or he may assign a specific chapter or journal entry for you. If you're working on your own, where should you begin? Although *The Healing Journey Through Menopause* is designed to be used in the sequence presented, the progression of chapters and journal entries is intended for women just beginning this passage through life. For those of you coming to the book at another point along your journey, you may decide to begin with a chapter that particularly interests you or meets your present needs. Since everyone moves at her own pace, there is no single "correct" way or order to emotionally move through menopause.

Although menopause signals the end of one life phase and the beginning of another, that change doesn't take place overnight. In fact, the physical, emotional, and spiritual changes usually take place over many years. The next chapter, "A Road Map for Understanding Menopause," will help you think about where you are now in this developmental process, physically, emotionally, and spiritually. However you choose to use this book, read Chapter 2 before continuing.

Making Yourself Comfortable

You may not be used to keeping a diary or journal, and perhaps you feel unsure of how to best start. First, regardless of which chapter or entry you start with, decide which conditions and environment will best support your journal writing. Here are a few suggestions that may help make the process more comfortable and productive for you:

- Set aside a regular schedule for working through your journal, preferably at a time of day when you're fresh and have the most energy.

- Take breaks during your writing if you need to. Stretching your legs can also give your mind a break.

- Think about the kind of environment that will best suit and support your writing. Would you prefer a brightly lit room filled with sunlight, or a room quietly lit by candles? Scents and smells might be an important environmental consideration also. Many people fill their writing environments with the fragrance of potpourri or incense. Consider playing some quiet music or other relaxing background sounds.

- For many, writing can be enhanced by a cup of soothing tea or a favorite drink, the comfort of a favorite chair or the feel of a comfortable piece of clothing.

- Pick a place to read and write that will be emotionally comfortable for you. Do you prefer a quiet private location or a public community area? If writing is emotionally difficult for you, or you find your feelings or thoughts overwhelming at times, consider having a comforting picture or object nearby or something else that might be familiar or emotionally safe.

- Make sure there's someone available for you to talk to after you write, if you think you may need some personal contact or support.

- Once you've completed an entry, reread it. Reflecting on what you've written can help you gain new insights.

Pick a place to read and write that will be emotionally comfortable for you.

Using the Entries

The styles for different journal entries in *The Healing Journey Through Menopause* vary, and each entry is provided only once. There are some entry formats that you may especially like using, and there are entries that you'll want to repeat more than once. Feel free to keep a *supplemental* journal in addition to this book where you can add your "spillover" thoughts or write additional entries. You may also want to photocopy certain blank entries in this book so that you can complete that entry more than once.

Each journal entry ends with a Things to Think About section, a series of questions for you to consider after you've completed your entry. These aren't a formal part of the entry but instead are reflective points that may spark a further journal entry, serve as discussion points if you're sharing your experience with a friend or counselor, or simply act as a focal point for your thoughts.

Sharing Your Experiences and Getting Help

Sometimes the act of writing about and exploring life can be uncomfortable. Working through some of the journal entries in this book may evoke difficult feelings because you're examining your own life, and looking back isn't always full of fond reminiscences. Looking back can remind you of those things that were good but also those things that weren't so good or that were outright painful. You may discover that unresolved feelings and unfinished business are often difficult to revisit, and even harder to settle. But you may also discover that taking stock of where you've been in your life can ease your way through menopause and increase your sense of anticipation and preparation for the next forty or fifty years of your life. If you find this process especially difficult, con-

Working through some of the journal entries in this book may evoke difficult feelings because you're examining your own life, and looking back isn't always full of fond reminiscences.

sider seeking help from a trained counselor or therapist, a menopause support group, or a physician or center that specializes in women and menopause.

Your Experience with Menopause

Menopause is a natural process. For some women the change is just not an issue. In fact, many women experience few physical problems with menopause and little in the way of emotional distress. Many women are never moved to reexamine their lives in light of menopause nor to assess their identity and relationships. However, some come to see menopause as not only a physical change in the life of an *individual* woman but also as a symbol of the way women have come to see themselves as a whole at this time in our history. In this view, menopause is seen as a celebration of womanhood. For other women, menopause represents a dramatic change in their bodies and self-image, sometimes accompanied by significant physical, emotional, and spiritual symptoms. Others still find that even though they are having little difficulty with this passage in their lives, they nevertheless feel that they *should* be more concerned. But the fact is there is no correct way to think about, experience, process, or deal with menopause. There's only *your* way. The significance given to menopause in your life is something that only you can assign. The bottom line is that menopause is experienced differently by different women.

Breathing Fresh Air

There are so many things going on in our fastpaced and highly stressed lives that we don't stop to think about this very moment. *The Healing Journey Through Menopause* will help you not only understand your life in the past, present, and future but will also

Although people often refer to breathing space as a metaphor for pause and examination, it's quite literally *important to find breathing space.*

provide the reflective and breathing space needed to make an assessment of your present life and determine your future.

Although people often refer to breathing space as a metaphor for pause and examination, it's quite *literally* important to find breathing space. Breathing and relaxation exercises can change both physical and mental states, affecting brain wave patterns and helping to relax muscles, and can even influence the capacity to learn. In their highly stressed lives, many people never stop to breathe deeply. As a result, lung capacity is never fully used nor blood fully oxygenated. Dozens of health books and health training disciplines recommend and describe breathing exercises as a source of good health and well-being. Andrew Weil, M.D., recommends that if you do no other exercise at all, ten deep breaths each day will be beneficial. Before continuing on to Chapter 2, take some time now to breathe deeply and completely, and then complete the following journal entry.

Take five deep breaths, clear your mind and let it wander while breathing, and physically and mentally relax for about five minutes before completing your entry. The relaxation is as important as the deep breathing it follows. Complete the entry in this relaxed state of mind.

A BREATH OF LIFE
1. Take your breaths, and then continue to relax for at least five minutes. Describe the experience.

_____

_____

_____

_____

_____

2. Complete these sentences.

a. *Breathing this way makes me feel* . . . _____

_____

_____

b. *With each breath, I* . . . _____

_____

_____

3. What thoughts or feelings ran through your mind as you breathed?

_____

_____

_____

_____

_____

4. What thoughts or feelings ran through your mind as you relaxed after the breathing exercise?

_____

_____

_____

_____

_____

5. Complete these sentences.

a. *Breathing this way opens me up to* . . . _____

_____

_____

b. *Breathing this way symbolizes my journey by* . . . _____

_____

_____

THINGS TO THINK ABOUT

- Do you usually stop to breathe deeply during your day? If not, what was it like to concentrate in this way, shutting out the things that perhaps normally distract you from your own body?
- Is this an entry worth repeating, perhaps even daily?
- What can deep breathing teach you about personal health care?

2

A Road Map for
Understanding Menopause

JANET

My first reaction going through "the change" was surprise. My mother hadn't told me about menopause, and though it's in all the books and on TV all the time, I kind of forgot it could happen to me too. I didn't know what to make of my first hot flash and thought I had a fever or someone had turned up the heat. After a while, I found myself wearing lighter-weight clothes and thought others were too warmly dressed. I woke frequently during the night, often with night sweats and sometimes with a fluttering heart. I couldn't get a good night's sleep and wasn't sure if my daytime irritability was due to interrupted sleep or some other reason. I read somewhere that night sweats were a symptom of tuberculosis, and for a while thought I might really be sick.

When I finally went to see my primary care physician he quickly eased my mind about TB, but he kind of ignored everything else. I asked about menopause, but he told me I was too young to be menopausal, and, besides, as I was still menstruating rather regularly I didn't have to worry about it. He even suggested that my physical symptoms were the result of a mild anxiety disorder. A good friend

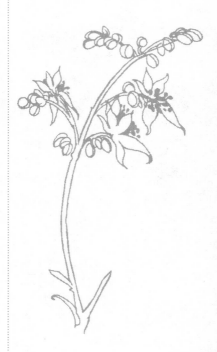

suggested I see someone who knew more about women's health issues. When I did, I began to realize I wasn't sick or crazy; I was peri-menopausal.

FOR ALL WOMEN, menopause is an important developmental milestone in their physiology. It also can be an important emotional, intellectual, and spiritual milestone. Women experience the changes brought about by the end of the ovaries' production of estrogen and progesterone in many different ways. As you're reading this book, you're probably looking for ways to make sense of this change and to figure out how to best understand, deal with, and work through it. Some women become aware of the signs of menopause and wonder what's happening to them without realizing that they've reached an important point in their lives. Others, like Jill in the introduction to this chapter, hardly notice a change. Still other women are thrust into menopause by a medical procedure.

As you're reading this book, you're probably looking for ways to make sense of this change and to figure out how best to understand, deal with, and work through it.

The first step to getting help is deciding whether you need any help in the first place. The second is knowing what kind of help is needed. Do you require, for example, medical treatment, personal education, lifestyle counseling, emotional support, or spiritual guidance?

Even though your experience of menopause will be unique, there are nevertheless some features typical of menopause in general. Understanding these will allow you to better recognize and understand your own experience and find your way along your journey. This process involves education about the *objective* realities, or the developmental and physical processes of menopause. Learning to tune in to your thoughts and feelings in a deliberate way and understanding your *subjective* experience is just as important.

Some cultures have developed traditions that allow for and encourage contemplation. For example, "moon lodges" were available for menstruating women to be away from daily life and contemplate the life-giving cycle. But we live in a culture that's short on rituals and celebrations for women beyond the childbearing years or for a general population that's aging. Journal writing can be your ritual, allowing a formal time and place to put aside other responsibilities and tend to yourself.

Although there's considerable discussion about menopause today, there are also many divergent opinions about the best course of action. Some believe that hormone therapy is all that's needed. Others support natural remedies, proven and improved over time and practice. Either way, whether hormone replacement therapy (HRT), naturalistic medicine, or physical exercise and meditation are part of your plan, they are only part of the picture. The larger picture is likely to involve not only your physical health but also seeing and experiencing yourself in a new way.

Journal writing can be your ritual, allowing a formal time and place to put aside other responsibilities and tend to yourself.

A New Frame of Reference

Menopause occurs over time and passes through several physical and emotional stages. Identifying and exploring your thoughts, feelings, and ideas as you enter and pass through each stage can be a real help in both figuring out what you need and where you are in this journey.

You'll most likely interpret the first signs of this change of life not as menopause or perimenopause, but as something else. You'll use whatever framework that has always helped you to make sense of your body and emotions up until now. For this reason, you may think your hot flashes or heart palpitations are signs of a physical illness, a panic attack, a mood swing, or premenstrual tension. Most people use their current frame of reference to make sense of their lives. This means that it probably didn't dawn on you right away that you were having a *normal* experience, not suffering from a problem.

Perimenopause

Perimenopause is the early stage of menopause that may last up to fifteen years. Your body begins and completes the developmental changes that culminate in menopause. The term *menopause* refers to the end of your menstrual periods: the prefix *meno-* means "menstruation" and *pause* means "stop." Often, physicians consider one year without periods as a confirming marker that menopause has been completed. During perimenopause (the prefix *peri-* means "around," as in "perimeter"), many hormonal changes take place. The average age at which women cease to menstruate is fifty-two, but your body may begin its developmental journey as early as age thirty-eight.

Because this change usually occurs over a period of many years, it gives you time to make sense of the physical, emotional, social, and spiritual shifts that occur. Many of the changes that occur at this time of life for women are the normal and expected signs of menopause, not symptoms of a problem. Your journal can assist you in becoming aware of and tracking these changes, reflecting on their impact and their meaning, and deciding how best to handle them.

As every woman is different, there's no way to define exactly how things will change for you. Often this natural stage of development begins as a change in your expected physical functioning. Menstrual periods that have been as regular as clockwork may become irregular, or usually light periods may become heavy. Moods may feel different too. Some women, for instance, describe feeling constantly premenstrual.

During perimenopause, your mind and body enter a different kind of dialogue, because although your ovaries are releasing fewer eggs and producing less estrogen and progesterone, your brain doesn't understand why the ovaries aren't doing their usual work. So it sends a messenger (follicle-stimulating hormone, or

During perimenopause (the prefix peri- *means "around," as in "perimeter"), many hormonal changes take place.*

FSH), which prompts the ovary to releases eggs. But this doesn't work if there aren't any eggs to be released. In fact, your ovaries don't actually *grow* eggs. Instead, they release eggs through follicles that were developed by your body in the first weeks of your life. As you reach menopause, there are fewer active follicles in the ovary; consequently, the FSH fails to do much. Because the brain doesn't realize this at first, it continues sending the FSH messenger. The fluctuation in hormone levels during this time—perimenopause—results in the following signs:

- hot flashes
- night sweats (a hot flash at night)
- interrupted sleep and insomnia
- headaches
- vaginal dryness
- urinary incontinence (some escape of urine when you laugh, for instance)
- weight gain around your midsection, where perhaps you've never gained weight before
- itchy, crawly skin and change in skin texture (such as dryness and wrinkles)
- changes in the pattern of your period (e.g., irregular or unusually heavy flow)
- fatigue
- joint aches and pains
- irritability and mood swings (the blues, temper outbursts)
- less interest in sex
- cognitive changes (e.g., lapses in short-term memory or problems with word retrieval)

Many of these natural signs of perimenopause can also be symptoms of medical or emotional problems, some of which may be serious. Any changes in how your body, emotions, or mind usually work are important to notice and check out. Persistent difficulty or special concerns with any of these changes should warrant particular attention. For this reason, it's important to check in with your primary care physician or a health care provider who can help you answer the question "Am I in perimenopause, or is this a problem of some kind that needs attention?"

Sudden Menopause

For some women menopause comes suddenly, however. Medical procedures such as partial or complete hysterectomy or ovarian radiation therapy can suddenly introduce menopause with the cessation of ovarian functioning. Here changes and adjustments that might have otherwise taken place over a period of many years are thrust on you. The problems of adjusting emotionally and physically to menopause are potentially increased under such conditions.

Life after Menopause: Stages of Awareness

Perimenopause, and then menopause, will run its own course. Although every woman will have a different experience with menopause, it's a natural process that follows a fairly predictable sequence of biological change.

Women also pass through emotional, intellectual, and spiritual changes. Changes of this sort usually don't happen all at once but instead evolve over time. Awareness passes through a set of developmental stages in which the gains of each stage build on the experience of the previous stage. For many women, the first stage is fairly predictable: an initially dim but then growing awareness that you've entered perimenopause. After this, different wo-men will have different experiences as they deal with and resolve their feelings about menopause. However, many women pass through a set of stages in which that first dim awareness becomes a building block for a physically and emotionally healthy life after menopause.

Just as there's no correct speed through which women pass through the physical aspects of menopause, there's no right or set pace for the development of personal awareness. Given how long the process of menopause can last, it's helpful to think of these as stages of emotional, intellectual, and spiritual awareness and growth that may take place over many years.

The signs of perimenopause will present themselves to you over time.

STAGE 1——BEGINNING AWARENESS: IS THIS REALLY PERIMENOPAUSE?

Prior to this time, you probably thought little about menopause in terms of its actual onset. For this reason, there's no clear "start" to this stage. Instead, the signs of perimenopause will pre-sent themselves to you over time. For instance:

- You experience physical and emotional changes that you can't explain through your usual frame of reference.
- Female friends of the same age are having similar experiences.
- You begin to notice media attention on menopause.

Focus of Attention

Because in many ways this is an entirely new experience, you may have few emotional and intellectual resources available to make clear sense of these changes in your body and mind. Your frame of reference hasn't yet begun to shift in order to accom-modate new information and make the emotional and cognitive adjustments required. Initial reactions will vary but are likely to include:

- surprise as you realize that menopause can happen to you
- denial because you *can't* believe that menopause *is* happening to you
- confusion about what your signs of change actually mean
- anxiety and fear about the changes that might follow (e.g., aging and mortality, personal attractiveness, changing relationships, or just the unknown)
- lack of control over a changing physical and emotional landscape

Task

During any stage of life, you encounter developmental tasks, which are things you have to do to get through menopause and pave the way for the next stage in your growth. In other words, you have to walk before you can run. Perhaps the most significant thing to accomplish during this important time is to question signs of physical and emotional change, and determine whether they signal perimenopause or some other condition you need to check out with your doctor. This will lay the groundwork for both health and personal growth.

Progress

From first noticing personal changes, you pass through a period of increasing awareness until you realize that you are in the perimenopausal phase of your life. Most likely, you're not sure of what this all means, but by the end of this first leg of your journey you're aware of and accepting that you're most likely experiencing perimenopause.

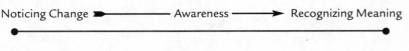

Noticing Change ➤——————— Awareness ————➤ Recognizing Meaning

Stage 1: Beginning Awareness

Developmental tasks are things you have to do to get through menopause and pave the way for the next stage in your growth.

STAGE 2—SHIFTING PERSPECTIVE: THIS IS PERIMENOPAUSE.

The time it will take you to pass through the first stage depends on the type of person you are. You may have realized you were entering perimenopause almost at once and quickly moved to this next stage where you begin to deal with the reality of being perimenopausal. The second stage of developing self-awareness most clearly begins when you get confirmation from your doctor that the signs you're experiencing are not due to an illness or other condition, and your attention begins to shift to your changing self.

Focus of Attention

During this early stage of personal awareness, your focus begins to change. Some women will be extremely internally focused, whereas others will barely notice any changes at all. Nevertheless, as awareness grows, so too does reflection. In this stage, the center of attention is turned inward to internal experiences. Tune in and ask yourself the following:

- What do I find myself talking to myself about?
- What's the nature of my "self" talk: constructive, neutral, or destructive?
- What's my attitude toward intervention and help and the vast options now available for intervention?
- What's my attitude toward my changing self?

Task

Listen to your body and learn about how you're changing. Pay attention to your thoughts, feelings, images, and ideas. Tune in to yourself, body, mind, and soul.

Progress

Awareness of perimenopause changes to a realization that you've entered this passage of your life. As you work through this second stage, your self-knowledge increases and you begin to acquire information about what resources are out there to help and whether you need any help at all. As you near the beginning of the third stage, you recognize that you must take charge of personal changes rather than simply allowing them to sweep you along.

Listen to your body and learn about how you're changing.

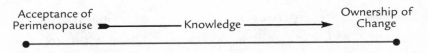

Acceptance of Perimenopause ➤————— Knowledge ————➤ Ownership of Change

Stage 2: Shifting Perspective

STAGE 3——FOCUSING ON SELF: WHAT'S BEST FOR YOUR BODY AND MIND?

In this third stage, your frame of reference is changing. You're aware that your body is going through changes that are the normal signs of perimenopause. Now the focus turns away from figuring out what's happening to you and more toward determining your specific needs. You realize that current health care decisions may affect you for the rest of your life, and you begin to think about what you need to do to take care of your physical, emotional, and spiritual health.

Focus of Attention

For many women, personal health issues until now have centered on a present medical need, such as an illness or birth control, or have involved someone else's health as well, such as pregnancy. No doubt this has begun to change somewhat as you've grown older, and you've already begun to pay more attention to long-term health risks, such as cancer and heart disease, and health enhancements, such as physical exercise and nutrition.

But facing menopause may be the first time you've started to make health care decisions strictly for yourself in the context of the rest of your life rather than the here and now.

- Think about the issues that are coming up in your life.
- Look at the themes you find in your thoughts, feelings, images, and ideas.

Task

Remember that women have never before had a longer post-menopausal life expectancy than they do now. Make decisions about what's best for your health over the long run and for the rest of your life.

Progress

The work of this stage begins with a focus on yourself. With increasing exploration you begin to learn more about yourself and your physical and emotional needs and well-being. Toward the end of the stage, your focus turns away from increasing self-discovery to a focus on what's out there that can really help you decide who you want to be and how you want to live your life.

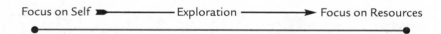

Focus on Self ➡━━━━━ Exploration ━━━━━➤ Focus on Resources

Stage 3: Focusing on Self

STAGE 4——FINDING WHAT'S GOOD: WHAT'S OUT THERE FOR YOU?

Of course, there's no end to personal development. Life and continued emotional and intellectual growth go on far beyond the completion of this fourth stage. In many ways the stage has no end. Instead, its completion is really marked by the realization that menopause has served as a springboard into the second half of your life.

Focus of Attention

Attention is largely directed toward getting and making sense of information and resources that are available to you. During this stage, you're not only dealing with issues of menopause, but you're also really preparing for life afterward. Consequently, the drive during this stage is to match resources, information, and help to personal needs and goals. This includes:

- figuring out where the resources are, and how to gather information
- learning how to interpret, sort out, and understand important information
- making sense of your own personal preferences about conventional versus alternative forms of help

You start this final stage with the determination to make decisions about what's best for your health and your lifestyle and to take charge of your own life.

Task

You recognize menopause as an important passage in your life, and a time for reflection and preparation. The task here is to assimilate what you've learned into a model for living your life both during menopause and beyond.

Progress

You start this final stage with the determination to make decisions about what's best for your health and your lifestyle and to take charge of your own life. At the other end is the sense that you've accomplished this goal. The decision to take charge has allowed you to determine how you live your own life.

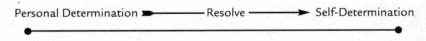

Personal Determination ➤——— Resolve ———➤ Self-Determination

Stage 4: Finding What's Good

Your Journey

Every woman will take a different path through menopause. Some women will negotiate the issues, the changes, and the bumps in the road smoothly. Some may not even notice the change or feel any physical or emotional discomfort. Others will struggle with health issues and other life changes. Still other women will use this time as an opportunity for introspection and renaissance. The goal for this chapter is to assist you in locating yourself along your particular journey, whatever route it may take. Use this next journal entry to think about where you are developmentally along your journey.

CHECKPOINT: STAGES

Based on the descriptions in the preceding pages, circle the letter that most closely describes your personal experiences.

	Not Yet Experiencing	Now Experiencing	Finished Experiencing
Stage 1 Experiences			
You're experiencing physical or emotional changes.	A	B	C
You can't explain these changes.	A	B	C
You're confused about what these changes mean.	A	B	C
You're wondering if this is menopause or an illness.	A	B	C
Stage 2 Experiences			
Your "self" talk has changed.	A	B	C
You're thinking about what change will mean and bring.	A	B	C
You're wondering if you need help with these changes.	A	B	C
You realize you're experiencing perimenopause.	A	B	C

	Not Yet Experiencing	Now Experiencing	Finished Experiencing
Stage 3 Experiences			
You're considering what's important in your life.	A	B	C
You're figuring out what these changes mean to you.	A	B	C
You're recognizing that decisions will affect your whole life.	A	B	C
You're thinking about what's best for your future.	A	B	C
Stage 4 Experiences			
You're assimilating what you've learned about your health.	A	B	C
You're making decisions about how to best live your life.	A	B	C
You're making decisions that will affect life after menopause.	A	B	C
You're ready to move on with the kind of life you want to lead.	A	B	C

Getting Located

You've now begun to think about stages of developing awareness and your own particular journey through menopause. Your Checkpoint journal entry helped you identify where you are with respect to each of these stages. Now look at the Checkpoint answers you've circled and complete the next entry.

WHERE ARE YOU?

1. Which task is most relevant to you *now*, in your current stage of awareness? Check one, or add a task that you feel is most important to you.

__determining whether physical or emotional changes are signs of menopause or symptoms of some other condition that you should check out with your doctor

__listening to your body and learning about how you're changing, as well as paying attention to your thoughts, feelings, images, and ideas.

___making decisions about what's best for your health over the long run and for the rest of your life.

___recognizing menopause as an important passage in your life, and assimilating what you've learned into a model for living your life both during menopause and beyond.

other: _____

2. What are your greatest concerns about menopause right now?

_____

_____

_____

_____

3. What are your current goals for dealing with or better understanding this time in your life?

_____

_____

_____

_____

4. What's your current stage in dealing with or understanding menopause?

___Stage 1—Beginning Awareness

___Stage 2—Shifting Perspective

___Stage 3—Focusing on Self

___Stage 4—Finding What's Good

5. Was it easy or difficult for you to easily identify your current stage? Why?

_____

_____

_____

_____

_____

6. Do these stages fit your own particular experience of menopause? If they do, how? If not, how is your experience different?

_____

_____

_____

_____

_____

_____

THINGS TO THINK ABOUT

- Does the idea that there are emotional and intellectual stages to the development of awareness in menopause fit your own experience? Is your experience less linear and more like a mosaic?
- If you have a spouse or children, how are their needs and concerns affecting you and your decision-making process? Have you been sharing with them enough about what's going on for you?

Using Your Feelings as a Guide

You now have a sense of your current stage and some of the issues you face and those that are yet to come. But menopause doesn't take place overnight. Although you may make personal decisions about health care and lifestyle changes, the emotional and developmental issues of change evolve slowly and over time. Although you can certainly influence and even speed up the process, there's no quick way to work through the emotional issues and life situations stimulated by menopause.

Without your intervention, the physical side of menopause will run its own course. Although you can't change the outcome of menopause (that is, you will stop ovulating), your intervention can nevertheless influence the way this change affects you. Your choice of an intervention is important because it reflects discrimination and self-determination. The interventions you choose may be physical, emotional, or spiritual in some way, or all three. Whatever your choices, they will be the result of your process of self-reflection, which involves sifting through and thinking about the mass of feelings you're experiencing and allowing yourself to describe and express them. "Feeling" emotions is one of the critical elements to any form of self-expression.

Not everyone likes their feelings, and not everyone wants to experience them. Some people try to avoid or squelch their overwhelming and perhaps negative feelings. Sometimes people don't even recognize that they're having feelings, or they don't realize the control their emotions have over their behavior. One goal of journal writing is to find ways to recognize feelings, accept difficult emotions, and learn to manage and work through them.

Although you can certainly influence and even speed up the process, there's no quick way to work through the emotional issues and life situations stimulated by menopause.

All feelings, even the ones you'd rather avoid, serve as a guide to what's going on inside you. Your feelings can help you gauge what's right and wrong for you and help guide your way. If you're in touch with your feelings they can help point to the issues that are affecting you and provide direction in how to best deal with these triggers. It's important to let them instruct and guide us, not control us.

The next journal entry asks you to think about current issues, concerns, or themes in your life. As you work through this entry, let your feelings guide your answers. This journal entry can also help you decide how best to use this book for yourself. By turning to the chapter number listed next to each item in parentheses, you can deal with issues that are particularly relevant now. If you want to work through this book sequentially, you may still want to come back to this list every now and then to see which issues are most pressing at any given time.

IDENTIFYING YOUR CONCERNS

1. Check off all the items that best describe what you're generally experiencing at this point in your life. (The numbers in parentheses next to each feeling indicate the chapters most relevant to dealing with that issue.)

ANXIOUS ABOUT:

___ aging (3, 4, 8, 11, 14)

___ changes in relationships (11, 12, 13)

___ changes in self-image (3, 4, 5, 9, 10)

___ changes in sexuality (5, 9, 12)

___ mortality (3, 4, 11, 14)

CONCERNED ABOUT:

___ difficulties in managing feelings (5, 6, 7)

___ emotional health (3, 5, 6, 7)

___ mood swings (3, 5, 6, 7)

___ onset of menopause (3, 4, 5, 6)

___ personal health (4, 5, 6)

___ physical changes (3, 6, 11)

CONFUSED ABOUT:

___ emotional changes (3, 5, 7)

___ lifestyle changes (5, 8, 9, 11, 14)

___ physical changes (3, 6, 11)

CONTEMPLATIVE ABOUT:

___ personal growth (8, 9, 10, 11, 14)

___ relationships (8, 9, 11, 12, 13)

___ the future (8, 11, 13, 14)

___ the past (5, 8, 11, 13)

___ the present (11, 12, 13)

EXCITED ABOUT:

___ changing times (5, 8, 9, 11, 14)

___ new ways of seeing things (9, 10, 14)

___ opportunities for personal growth (10, 13, 14)

___ possibilities for the future (13, 14)

LOST WITHOUT THE PREDICTABILITY OF:

___ monthly cycles (4, 5, 7, 9, 11)

___ familiar emotions (5, 7)

OVERWHELMED BY:

___ choices and decisions (10, 13, 14)

___ emotions (5, 6, 7)

___ responsibilities (4, 5, 11)

___ thoughts (4, 5, 7, 11)

SURPRISED BY:

___ the onset of perimenopause (3, 4, 5)

UNSURE OF:

___ health care choices (4, 5, 6)

___ how to tell if you're experiencing menopause (3, 4, 5, 6)

___ whether or not to consult a doctor (3, 4, 5, 6)

WORRIED ABOUT HOW THE CHANGES WILL AFFECT:

___ emotions (3, 5, 6, 7)

___ health and health needs (4, 5, 6)

___life in general (4, 5, 9, 10)

___lifestyle (5, 9, 11, 14)

___personal choices and freedom (9, 11, 12, 14)

___relationships (11, 12, 13)

___sexuality (5, 12)

2. Of the concerns you checked off, which four are most pressing right now?

_____   _____

_____   _____

THINGS TO THINK ABOUT

• Do you share your feelings with anyone else? If not, what stops you?

• Do your feelings seem so overwhelming at times that you need support? Who can you turn to for personal or professional help?

Charting Your Own Course

Menopause is a rich mixture of biological changes, psychological shifts, and adjustments in relationships. It's an experience both common and unique to every woman. Your history, present state of health, relationships, risk factors for illness, unfinished business, coping style, and wishes and vision for the future come together at this juncture in your life to define what this change will be like for you.

Women today are immersed and fully involved in multiple and major life responsibilities. Many women have taken the opportunity to attend college and graduate school, and they may have responsibilities to their jobs and careers. These and other life choices have delayed childbearing, and today it's not uncommon for a fifty-year-old woman to be tending to the needs of her young or teenage children and her parents as well as to her own needs.

Menopause is a rich mixture of biological changes, psychological shifts, and adjustments in relationships.

While your body may be saying, "Pay attention to me," family life and job responsibilities still demand your time and can easily create a conflict between the inward and contemplative process called for by menopause and the rigors of your daily life.

As you wrap up your work in this chapter, take a few moments to think and write about the journey that lies just ahead.

CHECKING IN WITH YOURSELF

1. What sort of competing demands on your time and energy might conflict with your need to take care of your changing personal needs?

_____

_____

_____

_____

2. Complete these sentences.

a. *As I complete this chapter, I feel like* . . . _____

_____

_____

_____

b. *Right now, I'd like to* . . . _____

_____

_____

_____

c. *Lately, I've been feeling like* . . . _____

_____

_____

_____

d. *My most important current task is* . . . _____

_____

_____

_____

e. *I feel like I most need to work on* . . . _____

_____

_____

_____

f. *This time in my life is important because* . . . _____

_____

_____

_____

THINGS TO THINK ABOUT

- Do you have a clear sense of the sort of issues, feelings, and tasks that you'll be facing as you work through your menopause?
- Are the concerns or problems you're experiencing so severe or debilitating that you need support and help from a friend, physician, or professional counselor?
- If you're married or in a committed relationship, are you sharing your concerns and experiences with your partner? Are you asking family members and friends for their opinions, ideas, and support as you make decisions about your life?

3

Destination:
FIRST GLIMPSES

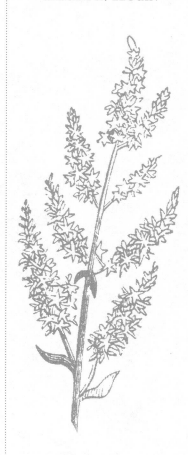

SANDY

At first I thought I was just having an "off" cycle. Then, each cycle was off in some way and it dawned on me that there was more going on than I'd initially thought. My body just wasn't doing what I was used to it doing. I didn't want it to change. I felt betrayed by my body, as though it were letting me down.

BETH

I remember being sort of concerned for at least a year before it dawned on me that I was entering menopause. I didn't worry too much, but I definitely didn't know what was going on when I felt my heart fluttering or had a hard time falling asleep at night. At first I thought I was having anxiety attacks because the symptoms matched those I'd read about, although I didn't feel anxious. It wasn't until I started getting hot flashes and my period became increasingly irregular that I started putting two and two together, and I began to realize that these signs meant the start of menopause, not some other unexplained problem with my mind or body. Even then it took a while to fully accept the idea that I was menopausal. I didn't feel old. I must

admit that although I took it in my stride, I did feel some concern
as I wondered what menopause was going to signal for my future.

MANY HAVE DESCRIBED the human life cycle and the stages of human development, with each stage dependent and building upon the stage it follows. For women, the onset of menopause clearly symbolizes midlife, or middle adulthood, which spans the middle thirties to the late fifties and early sixties. In fact, given expanding life expectancy, it's less and less clear when "old" age actually begins and "middle" age ends.

For women, the onset of menopause clearly symbolizes midlife, or middle adulthood.

The Beginning of the Middle

Both women and men go through midlife changes. The most objective way to describe middle adulthood is simply in terms of the years this period covers, but despite being brought on by the physical reality of encroaching years, the experience of midlife is usually quite *subjective*. The term *midlife crisis* is defined not by age parameters but rather by the personal experiences of those in middle age. The experience is one of self-image, not age. Midlife reflection and doubts center around many things—peoples' image of themselves, their expectations of what they "should" have achieved by now, their perceptions about their relationships with others and how others see them (including their perceptions about how they're seen by younger people), and often their sense that time is slipping away.

While middle adulthood can be defined simply in terms of years, the midlife *experience* is a combination of both age and subjective experience (how you feel). The experience of menopause, for example, encompasses both its physical realities with an emotional, intellectual, and spiritual dimension. It is not simply a change in physical functioning; it is a passage from one stage of life into another.

If midlife and the menopausal experience is in part a state of mind, what defines and shapes it? And how do you spot the beginning of the change and manage the transition? One goal of midlife adjustment concerns "wellness." Although at one time wellness simply meant a healthy body, it has now come to symbolize healthy body, mind, and spirit. It entails an overall sense of well-being. Based on the work of the John D. and Catherine T. MacArthur Foundation midlife development project, wellness can be defined by six characteristics:

The midlife experience is a combination of both age and subjective experience (how you feel).

1. *Self-acceptance.* This is a sense of personal satisfaction and a healthy self-image, regardless of the direction life has taken.

2. *Purpose.* This is a set of values and goals that give direction and lend meaning to life.

3. *Environmental mastery.* This is the ability to manage the tasks and demands of everyday life.

4. *Personal growth.* This is a sense of accomplishment, personal competency, and continued development.

5. *Positive relationships.* These are successful relationships that provide meaningful ties to the larger world.

6. *Autonomy.* This is a sense of independence and self-determination.

The tasks of midlife begin with the realization that these six aspects of wellness define and shape the middle years and serve as an important guide for your passage through menopause.

Dawning Awareness: Noticing Change

Menopausal changes are sometimes dramatic, but more often than not perimenopause is something that creeps up on you. It may begin with changes in your body that you feel but don't quite understand. Sometimes these physical changes may alarm you (like heart palpitations or sudden sweats). You may wonder what's wrong, or you may give it little thought. Around the same time, you may notice changes in emotions and moods and the way you seem to be thinking about and experiencing the world.

When our bodies and minds are working the way they always have, we tend not to notice them. We start to sit up and pay attention, though, when something changes. Your awareness of perimenopause comes when realization of these changes disturbs your usual experience of yourself and the way you normally "know" yourself. It's important, then, to be aware of changes and recognize them for what they are.

You may feel as though you're "not yourself" anymore, or others may tell you this very thing. You may begin to notice perimenopause through the experiences of friends or family members who are of the same age. Perhaps your attention is drawn to perimenopause because of a television show, a movie, or other media coverage, or perhaps the awareness of menopause dawns because of a surgical procedure or medical intervention such as radiation treatment or chemotherapy or removal of your ovaries. Whichever route to awareness you take, in the earliest days it will be important to think about whether the signs you've spotted in yourself are the normal signs of perimenopause or some other condition you need to check out with a physician or counselor. Thinking that the signs of perimenopause are indicators of an illness or a mental health problem will lead you down the wrong path. On the other hand, writing off the symptoms of a physical illness or mental health problem as early menopause can be equally detrimental.

Before you can explore and manage change, you must first notice it. The next two journal entries will take you on an inner exploration. The first will help you to take a look at your emotional and spiritual wellness. When faced with probing questions about

When our bodies and minds are working the way they always have, we tend not to notice them. We start to sit up and pay attention, though, when something changes.

our own lives—even when we ask them of ourselves—we some-times can back away from honest and meaningful answers. Try to be as honest with yourself as you can as you tackle and develop your journal and your journal-writing skills. Remember, you're having a conversation only with yourself, unless you choose to share your journal and your dialogue with someone else.

Try to be as honest with yourself as you can as you tackle and develop your journal and your journal-writing skills.

EMOTIONAL AND SPIRITUAL WELLNESS

1. Describe your sense of self-satisfaction.

_____

_____

_____

_____

_____

2. How positive is your self-image? Circle the number that comes closest to describing how you see yourself (1 = a negative self-image in which you feel pretty ineffective and incompetent; 5 = a positive self-image in which you feel capable and competent).

Negative Self-Image	**Positive Self-Image**
I see myself as really ineffective.	*I see myself as really effective.*

1   2   3   4   5

3. Explain your answer. How do you see yourself, and why?

_____

_____

_____

_____

_____

4. How do you feel about this time in your life? Circle the number that comes closest to describing your level of satisfaction with your life right now (1 = general dissatisfaction; 5 = a positive feeling about your life.

Dissatisfied   **Satisfied**

I'm very dissatisfied with my life.   *I'm very satisfied with my life.*

1   2   3   4   5

5. How do you feel about your accomplishments in life?

_____

_____

_____

_____

_____

_____

6. Do you feel a sense of mastery and competency in your daily life? Explain.

_____

_____

_____

_____

_____

_____

7. Do you feel in control of your life and where it's going?

_____

_____

_____

_____

_____

_____

8. Are you satisfied with your current relationships? Do they provide meaningful ties to the world around you?

_____

_____

_____

_____

_____

_____

THINGS TO THINK ABOUT

- On a emotional level, were these simple or difficult questions to answer? Were you honest with yourself in your answers?
- Did you find any of your answers difficult to accept? If so, why?
- What does this simple inventory tell you about yourself, your needs, and your desires at this time in your life? Should you return to this entry to complete it again in a few days or weeks?

The Trinity of Change: Body, Mind, and Spirit

Menopause is a passageway that involves change and affects you at three levels: mental, spiritual, and physical. Each describes a different aspect of who you are. The physical realm is perhaps most obvious because it involves actual changes in your biology. Distinguishing between your mental and your spiritual self may be less clear, however.

Our inner world is a combination of many forces, but our "mental" life involves emotions and thoughts. Emotions are your feelings, such as sadness, pleasure, anger, and happiness. Your thoughts involve your ideas and provide the means by which we can explore, understand, and manage our feelings. The spiritual world in this context involves neither a belief in spirits nor re-

Your spiritual beliefs refer to the sense of meaning you derive from your life and your world or to the meaning you inject into the world.

ligion. Rather, the word *spirit* here is used in the sense of "old school spirit" or the "spirit" of an idea. Your spiritual beliefs refer to the sense of meaning you derive from your life and your world or to the meaning you inject into the world.

What we do and how we express our inner world involves our physical actions — or those things we do with our bodies. Our behaviors are, in the end, not only those things we do but also those things by which we are judged by others and the means by which we mold and reshape our world. Our personal psychology is the result of these three interacting and often inseparable personal qualities. In the previous entry you focused on your emotional and spiritual sense of well-being. Use this next entry to think about signs of change in body, mind, and spirit.

CHANGES WITHIN

1. Check off those statements with which you agree, and add others below.

__ I'm experiencing increased physical discomfort.

__ I'm experiencing new or strange body sensations.

__ I'm noticing changes in the way my body works.

__ I've had increased physical pains.

__ My sexual interests are changing.

__ Physically, I don't feel like myself.

other: _____

_____

2. If you've experienced physical changes, describe your thoughts or concerns in more detail. _____

_____

_____

3. Check off those statements with which you agree, and add others below.

___I can't understand my own moods.   ___I feel more upbeat than usual.

___I feel as though no one understands me.   ___I get more easily upset or irritated.

___I feel like I've lost control of my feelings. ___I'm experiencing emotional fluctuations
                                               and mood swings.

other: _____

_____

_____

4. If you've experienced emotional changes, describe your thoughts or concerns in more detail.

_____

_____

_____

5. Check off those statements with which you agree, and add others below.

___I have concerns about my attractiveness.   ___I wonder more and more about the future.

___I question my achievements in life.   ___I'm more concerned about my age.

___I sometimes feel I have little left to give. ___My thinking is sometimes more "fuzzy."

___I wonder how I'm judged my others.   ___My memory isn't what it used to be.

other: _____

_____

_____

6. If you've experienced thinking changes, describe your thoughts and concerns in more detail.

_____

_____

_____

7. Check off those statements with which you agree, and add others below.

__I sometimes feel my age is a barrier.   __My life seems to have less meaning.

__I'm not sure where I'm going from here.   __Things once important seem less so.

__I'm noticing changes in my relation-   __Things once unimportant now seem
ships and interests.   important.

other: _____

_____

8. If you've experienced spiritual changes, describe your thoughts and concerns in more detail.

_____

_____

_____

_____

THINGS TO THINK ABOUT

- Are you experiencing change in some or all of these areas? If so, what do you think the changes signify?
- There are many reasons that people experience changes in body, mind, or spirit. Are there are other important factors in your life that could be responsible for any changes?
- Are you concerned about what the changes may mean?

Reactions to Change

By now it's clear that there have been some changes in your physical, emotional, and spiritual life, and it's possible that you've already identified them as premenopausal signs. People react to change in different ways. Some are surprised, others deny the reality of change, and still others are frightened by the prospect that things will be different now. Because change can't always be controlled, some people may feel disempowered. Other individuals will experience confusion and uncertainty about what change signifies or how to deal with it.

The goal in any emotional work is not to deny or dispel feelings, but instead to learn to identify and manage them. In dealing with change, like all other emotional work, the goal is not to eliminate change but instead to learn to identify and manage it. Interestingly, the Chinese written word for *crisis* is composed of two symbols. Together, these icons provide insight into the two possible faces of the crisis of change: one icon translates into "danger," and the other means "opportunity."

The goal is not to eliminate change but instead to learn to identify and manage it.

What's your typical response to change? How do you deal with it? Use this next entry to explore how you think about and respond to the changes life deals you.

RESPONDING TO CHANGE

1. Do you generally see change as a friend to be welcomed, a foe to be feared, or an uninvited guest to be tolerated? Is there some other way to better describe your feeling about change?

_____

_____

_____

_____

2. What most describes your typical emotional response to change? Add others below.

__aggravation	__anxiety	__depression	__frustration
__anger	__apprehension	__enthusiasm	__irritation
__annoyance	__concern	__excitement	__pleasure
__anticipation	__confusion	__fear	__thrill

other: _____   _____

_____   _____

3. How do you typically deal with change?

_____

_____

_____

_____

4. How do you become aware of and assess the impact of change on your life?

___I learn about the ways that this change might affect my life.

___I learn everything I can about the changes that are coming or have arrived.

___I listen to my body.

___I listen to my internal dialogues and thoughts.

___I pay attention to my dreams.

___I pay attention to my emotions.

___I talk to other people who are supportive and understanding.

___I talk to other people who have expertise and knowledge in this area.

___I talk to other people who have experienced similar changes.

other: _____

_____

_____

5. In what ways might the changes brought by menopause represent "danger?"

_____

_____

_____

6. In what ways does this change signal "opportunity"? Opportunity for what?

_____

_____

_____

7. How do you expect to deal with this change of life that's been thrust on you?

_____

_____

_____

_____

_____

_____

THINGS TO THINK ABOUT

- How do you cope with change? Are you satisfied with the way that you respond to or accept change?
- Is change something you feel you have any control over, or is it something that controls you?
- What has this entry taught you about yourself?

Expressing Yourself

Some people reflect on change in writing, others in music or art. Some individuals turn to meditation or quiet relaxation to inwardly examine personal changes. These are all methods aimed at suspending external pressure and making sense of daily life. Beyond reflection, however, lies self-expression. More than an act of contemplation, self-expression allows an active outlet for turning feelings and ideas into stress-relieving action. Through self-expression, we're able to think about and act on our world.

Your journal is an ideal tool for noting and reflecting on change. Use the final journal entry in this chapter to capture and describe your feelings and thoughts about this important time in your life.

CHECKPOINT: YOUR CHANGING SELF

1. If you were to take a photograph of your life at this time, what image would most capture the changes?

_____

_____

_____

2. What favorite quotation, verse, or poem best summarizes your feelings and experiences with change at this time?

_____

_____

_____

3. What scent or smell most reflects this time in your life?

_____

_____

_____

4. Is there a favorite piece of music that captures the flavor and emotion of this time in your life?

_____

_____

_____

5. Think about the images, words, scents, and sounds you chose. What do your choices tell you about your reactions to this time in your life?

_____

_____

_____

_____

6. Complete these sentences.

a. *As I complete this chapter, I feel like . . .* _____

_____

_____

b. *Right now, I'd like to . . .* _____

_____

_____

c. *My most important current task is . . .* _____

_____

_____

d. *I feel like I most need to work on . . .* _____

_____

_____

THINGS TO THINK ABOUT

- Are there specific questions you need to answer for yourself before continuing your work in this book?
- Do you have a clear sense of the sort of issues, feelings, and tasks that you'll be facing as you enter and work through this passage in your life?
- Have you decided how you can best use help as you enter and work through menopause? What sort of help? Do you know where to find the help and support you might need?

4

Destination:

ACCEPTANCE AND ADJUSTMENT

JANE

Somewhere along the way, in the midst of hot flashes, broken sleep, and unpredictable moods, I got sick and tired of being stoic. I began to think about the way I handled aches and pains and realized I was a silent but resentful sufferer.

I started to seek out advice and help when I felt I needed it. I learned to speak out loud about what was going on, to my husband, to my friends, and to my physician. I started reading books on menopause, checked out the Internet, and joined a women's support group. I could accept what was going on, but I wasn't going to let it get me down, just grin and bear it, or travel the journey alone. For the first time in my life, I let people know when things were difficult for me, how I felt, and what I needed. Although this "new" side of me was rather foreign at first, I began to enjoy sharing and couldn't imagine how I'd been so quiet for the last umpteen years of my life. I started feeling like a new woman.

MENOPAUSE IS NO longer viewed by our society as a change of life that signals the beginning of the end for a healthy woman. The

"Composing a life is a little like making a Middle Eastern pastry, in which the butter must be layered in by repeated folding, or like making a samurai sword, whose layers of differently tempered metal are folded over and over."
—MARY CATHERINE BATESON, from *Composing a Life*

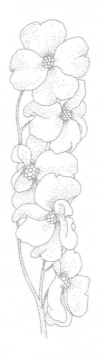

end of the childbearing years no longer indicates the end of a woman's value to society, nor does it imply imminent decrepitude or death. Instead, when we talk of a "change of life," we refer to exciting possibilities for personal growth and social contribution, not the withering away and drying up of a human life. The focus of this chapter is on your early entry into menopause and your acceptance of perimenopause and the start of this passage of change.

Meaning and Acceptance

The view of menopause as the end of youth, sensuality, and sexuality has now become outmoded.

As most people would probably prefer not to age, this journey in your life is most likely one you'd rather not begin. Menopause, however, is more than a journey of the body; it is also a journey of the mind. The meaning we give this passage reflects our own value system and our imagination. The view of menopause as the end of youth, sensuality, and sexuality has now become outmoded. Given that old interpretation, most women would not gladly accept menopause. And without acceptance, it's difficult to make adjustments and accommodations to a new phase of your life.

What does acceptance mean? First and foremost, it means acknowledging change and learning how to tolerate it. This is often not easy, and people develop many ways to avoid change or at least avoid dealing with it. Some people eat, drink, or drug themselves into a semicomatose reality so that they don't have to notice or be bothered by change. But all these behaviors simply serve to put off a successful adaptation to and acceptance of change.

Acceptance doesn't mean acquiescing or giving in. It doesn't mean liking or enjoying the new realities that may accompany a change. And it certainly doesn't mean becoming subservient to those new realities. Before you can accept change, though, you first have to recognize it. And to move beyond mere acceptance, you must be able to define (or redefine) change so that it serves, not represses, you.

Use this next journal entry to think about acceptance.

ACCEPTANCE

"Grant me the serenity to accept the things I cannot change, courage to change the things I can, and wisdom to know the difference."
——REINHOLD NIEBUHR

1. List four things that are difficult to accept during this time in your life.

a. _____

b. _____

c. _____

d. _____

2. Pick one of these items to focus on for the remainder of this entry, and describe why you chose it.

_____

_____

_____

_____

_____

3. What is the most difficult thing to accept about this time in your life?

_____

_____

_____

_____

_____

4. What does this thing represent for you?

_____

_____

_____

_____

_____

5. What is it like to have to accept this reality in your life?

_____

_____

_____

_____

_____

6. Is there a way to reframe this part of your life so that it's easier to accept?

_____

_____

_____

_____

_____

7. Review the verse that opens this entry. Is this a thing you *can* change, or a thing you *can't* change?

_____

_____

_____

_____

_____

Adjustment

Where acceptance requires an *acknowledgment* of the situation and the ability to assimilate the idea of change, adjustment is based on your ability to *adapt* to and *accommodate* the situation. Neither acceptance nor adjustment means you must like the situation, but both entail your ability to "roll with the punches." In the case of menopause, adjustment means both adapting to physical changes and accommodating a changing self-image. Mastery of change comes only after acceptance and adjustment.

Some people are able to adjust to change easily, and some aren't able to adjust at all. Adjustment isn't really a "thing" that you do, though; rather, it's a process that involves several components.

- *Acknowledging* that change has happened is the first requirement of adjustment. People who are in denial of the facts or unable to acknowledge what's happened or how they're feeling face great difficulty transitioning to this new part of their life.

- *Accommodation* means accepting the change into your life. It doesn't mean welcoming, liking, or agreeing with change; it simply means acclimating yourself and getting accustomed to the new reality. Those who constantly lash out angrily or

Adapting means making the necessary changes in yourself to work with and survive change in your environment.

can't get used to changes or disruptions to their lives are likely to experience ongoing discomfort and disappointment, and it will be difficult for them to find ways to make use of this experience.

◆ *Adapting* is key to survival. Adapting means making the necessary changes in yourself to work with and survive change in your environment. Those unable to change themselves to fit new circumstances may not prove resilient enough to meet the challenges of the world that has changed around them.

Use the next journal entry to think about adjustment and how you're dealing with each of these different elements.

ACKNOWLEDGMENT, ACCOMMODATION, AND ADAPTATION

1. Check off those areas you're adjusting to.

___changes in relationships   ___changes in the way you feel

___changes in self-image   ___changes in the way your body looks

___changes in the way others see you   ___changes in the way your body works

___changes in the way you experience life   ___changes in your thinking

other: _____   _____

_____   _____

_____   _____

_____   _____

2. Is there any question for you about the reality or permanence of these changes?

_____

_____

_____

_____

3. Do you doubt that the changes you're experiencing are related to menopause?

_____

_____

_____

4. Have you acknowledged the facts, or are you still at some level of denial?

_____

_____

_____

_____

5. Have you accepted the reality of these changes? Have you been able to acclimate yourself to them?

_____

_____

_____

_____

6. Have you been able to adapt to the changes, or are you fighting the changing of your life in some way?

_____

_____

_____

_____

7. Is there something you can do to better accommodate these changes or to help your process of acceptance and adjustment?

_____

_____

_____

_____

Personal Style and Adjustment

Your ability to adjust well to significant change is important. But it isn't as simple as just making up your mind to adjust and then getting on with it. Adjustment is both something that *you do* and something that happens *to you*. In the former, you make the appropriate changes in your behavior and attitude in response to an external situation. In the latter, you undergo a psychological change that allows you to operate effectively within the new situation. It's this second aspect of adjustment that's so critical. Without *internal* flexibility, it is difficult to accept or make *external* change.

Without internal *flexibility, it is difficult to accept or make* external *change.*

Personal adjustment can certainly be encouraged and fostered through supportive relationships and counseling. Nevertheless, adjustment is a task influenced by the interplay of four underlying personal factors.

1. *Psychological processes*. This process refers to the way you feel and think about and experience the world, both consciously and unconsciously. Your ability to adjust is tied to your ability to understand and, if necessary, change the way you think.

2. *Emotional connections*. These connections are the relationships you form with people and things and the way these re-

lationship bonds affect you. Adjustment usually means disconnecting from those emotional ties that limit and hold you back and developing emotionally satisfying connections that help you move toward your goals.

3. *Flexibility*. Flexibility is your ability to "roll with the punches." Adjustment is built on the ability to recognize and adapt to changes in the environment and is reflected in a lifestyle that has been redesigned to accommodate these changes.

4. *Integrative skills*. This skill refers to your ability to develop and live a life in which you've accommodated and incorporated change. As a result, you are able to exert more control over the way you live your life. The key lies in being able to integrate your experiences, using them as the basis for a new perception of reality—or the renewal of your life.

At this point in your life, the issues really aren't about *whether* to change or *why* you should have to change. The current task concerns *how* to change and identifying anything that might interfere with your ability to adapt to the changes you're experiencing.

EXPLORING ADJUSTMENT

"A tree that is unbending is easily broken.
The hard and strong will fall.
The soft and weak will overcome."
——LAO TSU

1. What difficulties do you typically experience with change and adjustment?

_____

_____

_____

_____

2. Complete these sentences.

a. *Three things most interfering with my ability to adjust are . . .*

_____

_____

_____

b. *Some things I can do to help me get over these hurdles to adjustment are . . .*

_____

_____

_____

THINGS TO THINK ABOUT

- Are you able to recognize circumstances or personal attributes that are affecting your ability to adjust? Have you learned anything surprising about yourself?
- Are you able to identify any specific ways to deal more effectively with adjustment problems?
- How important is it that you learn to accommodate these changes?

Talking to Yourself

What does change mean to you, and how do you typically react to it? Answering this question, of course, requires that you talk to yourself. In fact, people talk to themselves all the time. We call this process the internal dialogue. One of the things that a journal can do is bring these inner conversations into the world outside your head and onto paper where you can look at and think about what it is that's going on in your life.

Sometimes internal dialogue is healthy, involving a process in which your self-talk can help put things into a useful perspective, help make sense of the world, and boost your self-esteem. Other times, self-dialogue is neutral and has no impact one way or another. But for many people this inner talk can be negative and self-defeating. If you are full of self-doubt, or perhaps self-loathing, the dialogue will only serve to tear you down. Often built on irrational thoughts and ideas, a destructive internal conversation fosters an environment in which you become your greatest critic and your own worst enemy.

One way in which people think about, plan for, and deal with change is through their self-talk. Use this next entry to think about and explore your style of internal dialogue.

TALKING TO YOURSELF

1. What do you talk to yourself about? Is your self-talk positive and constructive, negative and destructive, or neutral?

_____

_____

_____

_____

_____

_____

_____

_____

2. What effect does your self-talk have on you? Does it help or hinder?

_____

_____

_____

_____

_____

3. Is your thinking about menopause rational and clear, or are your thoughts clouded by irrational fears and concerns?

_____

_____

_____

_____

4. What might help your self-talk to be more constructive and positive?

_____

_____

_____

_____

5. What can you do to decrease self-talk that is negative and overly self-critical?

_____

_____

_____

_____

THINGS TO THINK ABOUT

- Is it difficult to get in touch with and listen to you own self-talk? Is it useful to listen to yourself? Is it important?
- Does your self-talk need to change? What can you learn from your self-talk about what's important at this time in your life?
- Some people try to "quiet down" their internal dialogue. How might you go about this?

Where to from Here?

By now, you have a clearer sense of menopause and have measured your own point along this path. Ahead are decisions to be made, some of which may involve interventions designed to ease you through this major life change. These decisions may be aimed at your physical health and well-being or your emotional condition or lifestyle and personal growth.

The next journal entry will help you think about the steps you may need to take in terms of actual health decisions and with respect to your attitude toward your changing body and your health.

DECISIONS AND ATTITUDES ABOUT DECISIONS

1. How will you make decisions about your physical health? Check off all choices that fit for you, and add more below.

___ I'll discuss my concerns and medical issues with my current medical practitioner.

___ I'll discuss the issues and my concerns with family and friends, and seek direction there.

___ I'll gather as much information as possible and figure things out before taking any action.

___ I'll seek out a health practitioner who specializes in menopause or one who is recommended.

___ I'll use the Internet to discover sources of information and support.

___ I'll wait and see how things develop.

other: _____

_____

_____

_____

2. Describe your thoughts on seeking medical or health advice.

_____

_____

_____

_____

3. What attitudes do you hold about health interventions?

__I haven't made my mind up.

__I prefer alternative sources for the support and treatment of menopause, such as vitamins, diet, exercise, and meditation.

__I prefer conventional medical interventions.

__I prefer to deal with this as a completely normal process and let nature take its own course with no interventions at all.

__I prefer to handle as much as possible on my own, with as little intervention as possible.

__My attitudes are different at different times and under different circumstances.

other: _____

_____

4. Briefly describe your thoughts on preferred interventions.

_____

_____

_____

_____

5. How would you describe your emotional response to these physical changes?

__anxious   __confused   __excited   __grateful

__comforted   __disappointed   __frightened   __pleased

other: _____   _____

_____   _____

6. Write a few words describing how you're feeling about this change in your life.

_____

_____

_____

7. Check off those statements that describe your attitude toward your changing self, and add others below.

__I dislike these bodily changes.

__I feel a new freedom.

__I feel great about the naturalness of this change in my body.

__I feel let down by my body.

__I like these bodily changes.

__I miss the predictability and rhythm of monthly cycles.

__I'm anxious abut what other bodily changes may be ahead.

__I'm concerned about physical attractiveness.

__I'm excited about the change.

__I'm looking forward to creating new rhythms.

other: _____

_____

_____

_____

THINGS TO THINK ABOUT

- What have you learned from this journal entry about your attitude toward menopause?
- Do you feel you need some medical advice? Are you ready to seek medical advice?
- Are you emotionally prepared for this journey? If not, and even if you are, how can you further prepare yourself?

The Power of Self-Expression

Writing is a powerful tool for outlining your ideas, exploring your emotions, and expressing both.

The Italian playwright Ugo Betti wrote, "Thought itself needs words. It runs on them like a long wire. And if it loses the habit of words, little by little it becomes shapeless, somber." If it serves no other purpose, your journal is an outlet for *your* thoughts and feelings. Writing is a powerful tool for outlining your ideas, exploring your emotions, and expressing both.

Why does self-expression help? If unrelieved (or unexpressed), feelings often build up inside of people. Sometimes if held inside and unexpressed, difficult to manage feelings can contribute to depression, anxiety, and insecurity. They can eat away at you, and many believe they contribute to physical illness such as migraine headaches, stomach problems, and heart attacks. Emotions can also build up internal pressure until they explode outward in a fit of rage, an act of aggression, or some other external display of emotion. Whether feelings are turned inward or outward, few would consider these forms of expression productive or effective. When handled this way, suppressed emotions often become personally destructive rather than serving as a guide for self-exploration and personal growth.

Self-expression is the opposite of emotional suppression. It provides a means for appropriate and healthy emotional and intellectual venting. By putting your feelings and thoughts into words, you give shape and meaning to them. Self-expression connects you to your environment and the people in your life. But it doesn't only transform internal pressure; it also transforms *you*. Talking about a difficult situation won't change it, but talking can help you see things differently, relieve the pressure of the situation, and feel less emotionally entangled.

You've had the opportunity now to sit with yourself and your journal, listening to your body, your feelings, and your thoughts. As you reach the end of this chapter you've begun to recognize and note your attitude toward your changing self. Sometimes this work may stir up a host of positive and negative feelings. You may sometimes feel that the "old" you is in tune with the new and evolving you. At other times, you may feel nothing but conflict among the person you were, the person you are, and the person you're going to be.

By putting your feelings and thoughts into words, you give shape and meaning to them.

Use the last entry in this chapter to check in with yourself and to think about change in your life.

CHECKPOINT: THE CHANGING YOU

1. What kind of person are you?

_____

_____

_____

_____

_____

_____

_____

_____

2. Describe the personal changes you're going through.

_____

_____

_____

_____

_____

_____

_____

3. How are these changes altering and affecting the person you are?

_____

_____

_____

_____

_____

4. What kind of person would you like to be?

_____

_____

_____

_____

_____

5. How can these changes help you to become the person you'd like to be?

_____

_____

_____

_____

_____

_____

THINGS TO THINK ABOUT

- Have there been changes this dramatic or tumultuous at other times in your life? How does this time in your life compare with other important passages you've experienced?
- Have you thought of your life as a series of passages before now? Where are these "passages" leading?
- Are you okay with the change in your life, or are you fighting it every step of the way? Either way, how is your attitude affecting your ability to handle the change?

5

Destination:

KEEPING PERSPECTIVE ON YOUR MENOPAUSE

ELIZABETH

When I first realized I was entering menopause I experienced a lot of different feelings that I really couldn't sort out at first. I worried about aging and what it meant, I was definitely concerned about sexuality, and I wondered what this would mean for my health. I actually felt lost and really didn't know who to talk to about it—or even what to talk about.

I started reading books and watching TV talk shows. I read about women's health, different approaches to working with menopause, women's issues, and, with great interest, I read about the ideas, experiences, and stories of other women who had all gone through exactly the same thing I was going through right now. I started out with no point of view at all, but wound up with a perspective of my own. I was able to understand and put menopause into its place in my life. Now I don't have any trouble at all with the idea, although I'm still not exactly sure where it all leads.

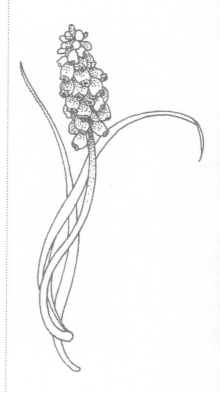

OFTEN IT IS our perspective, or our view of the world, that determines the facts, not the facts themselves. For this reason, it's important to gain a perspective on menopause that can help you both to locate yourself right now on your journey and to see the path ahead.

Where the *physical* reality of menopause is basically unaltered, its personal and social significance and meaning has changed dramatically. As more women are approaching or are in menopause, more now than ever are also fully in the grip of major life responsibilities. Women have taken the opportunity for furthering their education, devoting more time to career development, and have delayed bearing children. With an increasing life span, it's quite common for a fifty-year-old woman to be tending to the needs of her parents and her children as well as her own life outside the traditionally defined responsibilities. The fact that menopause takes place when women are still in the prime of their lives, still experiencing active responsibilities as parents and care providers, and perhaps still in the middle or beginning of a developing career or set of life interests is a dramatic departure from the former image of the menopausal woman as having reached the end of her productive life.

This chapter will help you gain perspective about menopause and its place in your life. Before you decide who you want to be and how you want menopause to affect and influence you, you have to decide what menopause means to you.

Getting a Perspective

"Perspective" is often tied up with attitude or mental outlook. For the most part, it means keeping things in proportion and seeing the *whole* picture even though your view may be distorted by circumstances. Developing a perspective often means getting an education about what's happening *now,* and what's likely to hap-

"Perspective" means keeping things in proportion and seeing the whole *picture even though your view may be distorted by circumstances.*

pen in the *future*. Quite frequently, this means looking "sideways" to the experiences of other women and looking "backward" into the history of the change and how it has affected and been seen by others. One way to gain a perspective is to examine the ideas of other people, which helps you develop your own ideas. The Internet alone provides a wealth of information, interaction, and communication. It offers updated medical and health information, the personal experiences and ideas of both health practitioners and women experiencing menopause, and is a gathering place for people who want to talk to one another about menopause. Health magazines and medical journals provide the latest theories and relevant studies; in addition, there are myriad books, radio programs, and television talk shows that explore the topic of menopause. In short, there are numerous sources that can help you to develop your own perspective.

Health magazines and medical journals provide the latest theories and relevant studies; in addition, there are myriad books, radio programs, and television talk shows that explore the topic of menopause.

These sources of information and ideas also provide different frameworks for developing your own perspective. Although many of these frameworks overlap with one another, perspectives on menopause can be categorized in the following ways:

- *Medical.* This perspective concentrates on the medical meaning, development, and treatment of menopause.

- *Health.* This point of view can be broader than the medical category, or it may not focus at all on a medical perspective, instead concentrating on nonmedical interventions such as diet and nutrition, exercise, and herbal remedies, for example.

- *Philosophical.* This predominant perspective entails a thought-provoking examination of the meaning and experience of menopause.

- *Anecdotal.* The stories and various experiences of other women who are entering or have passed through menopause provide the focal point.

- *Sociological*. This approach explores how menopause has been defined, understood, and incorporated into a larger social and cultural point of view.

- *Political*. The predominant ideas about menopause are examined or presented have controlled or dominated the lives of women.

- *Spiritual*. In this perspective the focus is on personal meaning, self-growth, and connections to a larger, more meaningful experience.

Developing a perspective without understanding the point of view of others is like learning to paint without studying the work of other artists or becoming a writer of fiction without reading other literature. Of course, you *can* do it, but your viewpoint will always be limited to just your own imagination and knowledge.

Perspectives on Health

One way to learn more about the medical and health aspects of menopause is to read the research, but it's important to have a sense of what kind of information you're looking for and an idea of how to make sense of the information. Because there are so many studies, information about interventions can be confusing and contradictory, and it is sometimes misused to sell products or promote a particular point of view. Before accepting its conclusion or recommendations lock, stock, and barrel, learn what you can about the study itself. Many of the books, articles, and other materials on menopause deal less with facts about the physical course of menopause than with interventions of one kind or another. Some factors to consider in choosing research material include the length of the article or study, the characteristics of the study group, the sponsoring organization, and the reputation of the research group.

Expanding Your Perspective

If you've been reading or studying about menopause, it will be important to stop and think about what you're learning, or more accurately, about what you're *thinking*. Use this journal entry to reflect on and think about what you're reading or studying.

DEVELOPING A PERSPECTIVE

1. What is the general theme of the material you've been reading or studying?

_____

_____

_____

2. What sort of perspective does it most seem to provide? Check all that apply, but mark the primary perspective with the letter *P*.

___health   ___medical   ___philosophical   ___sociological

___interventions   ___personal experience   ___political   ___spiritual

other: _____

3. Are the materials or ideas presented in this work mainly designed to give you information or facts, or are they designed to affect the way you *think* about menopause?

_____

_____

_____

4. Do the ideas presented interest you or seem relevant? If so, why? If not, why not?

_____

_____

_____

_____

5. What have you learned from this material?

_____

_____

_____

6. Are these ideas that you can incorporate into your own thinking?

_____

_____

_____

7. How do the facts or ideas presented help you to shape your own thinking and develop your own perspective?

_____

_____

_____

8. Do you feel a need to read more material like this?

_____

_____

_____

9. Are there other perspectives you feel a need to learn more about?

_____

_____

_____

THINGS TO THINK ABOUT

- Is it useful to stop and think and write about what you're reading before reading more? Is this sort of journal entry useful to you?
- Is the material on menopause you're reading or studying meeting your needs to learn more about menopause? Are you studying about the sort of things you really want to know about?

Checking in on Your Point of View

The previous journal entry provided a way for you to think about and reflect on the materials you're reading to learn about menopause and its possible (or actual) impact on your life. In some cases, perspective forms only after reading and hearing a great deal about a subject, but in other cases our opinions form quickly and aren't easily changed or shaped by the thoughts of other people. Take a few minutes now to think about your current point of view about menopause.

The next journal entry will allow you to start thinking and writing about your own perspective. At this point, your point of view may be well formed or barely developed. At whichever end of the spectrum your current perspective lies, like anything else, it may change over time. For this reason, this is an entry to revisit over time as your knowledge and perspective grows and changes.

EXAMINING YOUR PERSPECTIVE

1. What's your perspective about the physical processes involved in menopause?

_____

_____

_____

_____

_____

_____

2. Describe your thoughts on menopause and personal spirituality: its impact on self-image, relationships, and a generally larger sense of connection.

_____

_____

_____

_____

_____

3. What's your point of view regarding the role of treatment, remedies, or interventions?

_____

_____

_____

_____

_____

4. Do you have a point of view about interventions in your own life? Explain.

_____

_____

_____

_____

_____

_____

5. How will you decide about personal interventions?

_____

_____

_____

_____

6. Do you feel your perspective needs to be broadened?

_____

_____

_____

_____

_____

_____

_____

7. In what areas are your views on menopause the most clearly formed?

_____

_____

_____

_____

_____

_____

8. In which areas do you feel you need to learn more about the process of meno-pause?

__alternative medicine   __medical treatment   __political impact

__alternative lifestyle   __natural remedies   __research findings

__cultural significance   __nutrition and diet   __social history

__emotional impact   __philosophical   __spiritual significance

__health interventions   __physical process   __stories of other women

other: _____

_____

9. Generally describe your current perspective on menopause.

_____

_____

_____

_____

THINGS TO THINK ABOUT

- How well formed are your opinions about menopause? Do you think you have an open mind to different ideas, or is your mind already made up? Is it possible to have *too* much of an open mind?
- Do you need to read and learn more about the various aspects of menopause, or do you feel you already have enough information?
- Are you comfortable enough with what you already know about menopause to decide how best to proceed? If not, how will you go about learning more?

Keeping Perspective

Maintaining a perspective means seeing things broadly, with all the pieces on the table.

When people refer to "keeping perspective," they often mean seeing things clearly and maintaining a calm and focused attitude toward a perhaps unsettling, confusing, or chaotic time. In this context, maintaining a perspective means seeing things broadly, with all the pieces on the table. It means not letting your concerns, fears, anxieties, and perhaps even preconceptions about menopause take over. The goal is to sift through the available material and ideas as best you can, think about and explore their meaning, and base your decisions on a perspective that can help you move forward instead of holding you back.

One way to develop and keep a healthy, helpful perspective is to complete "reality" checks. Use the next journal entry to think about your perspective on menopause and how menopause will affect, or has already affected, your life.

SEEING CLEARLY

1. Will menopause . . .

___have a minor or a major effect on your functioning?

___leave you physically impaired?

___leave you emotionally impaired?

___leave you spiritually impaired, or without beliefs and meaning?

___change or strip you of the thing that makes you "you?"

other: _____

_____

2. Does your ability to reproduce govern your entire being, defining who you are?

_____

_____

_____

3. Do you think aging will limit your ability to grow emotionally, intellectually, and spiritually? Why or why not?

_____

_____

_____

4. Do you think menopause will affect the way you love or the way others love you? Why or why not?

_____

_____

_____

5. Do you feel menopause is a transition to the "end" of your life? How so?

_____

_____

_____

6. How will menopause change the quality of your life?

_____

_____

7. Are you giving up something as you enter menopause? If so, giving up what?

_____

_____

_____

_____

8. What does it mean to be menopausal?

_____

_____

_____

_____

THINGS TO THINK ABOUT

- Do you have fears about menopause? If so, are they well founded?
- Is your perspective on menopause a helpful one? Can it help move you forward, or might it hold you back in some way?
- What are your worst fears about menopause? How can you best address and overcome them?

Perspective from Inspiration

Perspective doesn't always come from the facts, or even from your experience. Sometimes perspective is the result of a flash of inspiration, a suddenly clear vision of the world. People sometimes refer to this sort of perspective and knowledge as the "aha!" experience because clarity and vision come suddenly and unexpectedly.

Art in all its forms can be a source for both inspiration and for developing a perspective. The simple images and ideas conveyed in a story, a painting, or a poem, for example, can serve to quickly expand our perspective if only we are open to new ideas and new ways of seeing.

There are many different formats for journal entries. The next entry is unstructured and free-form style. That is, it provides minimal instructions and requires that you complete the entry entirely in your own words and in your own way. One way to complete an entry like this is to think carefully about the question and write your answer only after some deliberation. Another way, often recommended in free-form writing, is to simply answer the question without too much thought, writing whatever comes to mind. There are no correct answers. This journal entry is based on the quotation that opens it. Use the brief verse as a guide to stimulate your own thoughts.

EVOKING PERSPECTIVE

"A road that does not lead to other roads always has to be retraced, unless the traveler chooses to rust at the end of it."
—TEHYI HSIEH

1. What image is evoked by this quotation?

_____

_____

_____

_____

_____

_____

2. What does this verse mean to you?

_____

_____

_____

_____

_____

3. What thoughts or ideas does this verse stimulate for you?

_____

_____

_____

_____

_____

4. How can this verse help you put your passage through life into perspective?

_____

_____

_____

_____

_____

THINGS TO THINK ABOUT

- Was this a difficult or easy journal entry for you to complete? Do you prefer structured or free-form journal entries?
- Did the verse selected for the entry "work" for you? Did it help you to place a perspective on your own journey? Are there other favorite verses or quotations that can help provide you with direction or stimulate perspective?

Creating Meaning

Perspective is related to meaning. Applying a particular perspective to a situation can allow you to make sense of and understand it in a way that might otherwise be impossible if seen from another angle. Much of your journey through this life passage is about just that. Applying a perspective may or may not alter the *physical* reality of menopause (which *can* change, for example, if your perspective includes HRT), but it can alter the *psychology* of menopause.

Your journey is still fresh, and there are many roads ahead. You probably still have many questions unanswered or even unasked. But by now you are beginning to see that it is possible to make meaning out of a jumble of bits and pieces. Sometimes, as you take seemingly disconnected parts and connect them, you *create* meaning. But it's only after you've built the connective links and created something new that you're able to look for the meaning within.

In the next entry, you're going to create a "fridge poem." The entry is named for the magnetic poetry kits for a refrigerator, which have recently become popular. These kits are made up of hundreds of individual magnetized words that are used to create messages or poems on your refrigerator, by arranging them in any desired order.

For this entry you can buy a fridge poetry kit or simply cut out a hundred words at random from any magazine. Whether you use a kit or cut out your own words, select between thirty-five and fifty of the words you've gathered, and create a poem inspired by your change of life.

Sometimes, as you take seemingly disconnected parts and connect them, you create meaning.

A FRIDGE POEM

1. After you've completed your fridge magnet poem, reproduce it here.

_____

_____

_____

_____

_____

_____

_____

_____

_____

_____

2. Reread your poem. How does rereading it make you *feel*?

_____

_____

_____

_____

3. What does rereading your poem make you *think*?

_____

_____

_____

_____

4. What meaning is there in this poem for you?

_____

_____

_____

_____

_____

_____

_____

_____

THINGS TO THINK ABOUT

- What's the difference between *making* meaning and *finding* meaning? Did you make meaning from, or find it within, the words you chose for your poem?
- Do you have to look for meaning to find it? How can you keep finding meaning?
- In Questions 2 and 3, were you easily able to distinguish between the way you feel and the things you think?

Existentialism

People often comment that life is what you make it. This is the essence of the philosophy of existentialism, or the idea that *we* determine who we are and who we're going to be. Søren Kierkegaard, sometimes considered the founder of existentialism, wrote in his journal, "I must find a truth that is true *for me.*" Do you agree with this sentiment? As you move through your journey, deeper into the second stage of this passage and toward Stage 3, this is an important time for perspective. To some degree, your perspective determines not only your emotional and spiritual experience with menopause (and perhaps your physical experience) but also the shape of your life as it unfolds ahead of you. Use the final entry in this chapter to reflect on who you are and how menopause can, should, or will shape that perceived self-image.

CHECKPOINT: ON BEING A WOMAN

1. Is there more to being a woman than the experience of childbirth?

_____

_____

_____

_____

_____

2. What lies beyond motherhood?

_____

_____

_____

_____

3. What *does* it mean to be a woman?

_____

_____

_____

_____

_____

_____

4. If married or in a committed relationship, what is your partner's perception of womanhood?

_____

_____

_____

_____

_____

5. What lies beyond marriage or other forms of committed relationships?

_____

_____

_____

_____

_____

6. What lies beyond romance?

_____

_____

_____

_____

_____

7. What lies beyond menopause?

_____

_____

_____

_____

_____

_____

8. What is menopause a passageway to?

_____

_____

_____

_____

_____

THINGS TO THINK ABOUT

- Is your role in society shaped or impaired in some way by becoming menopausal?
- Have the questions in this entry helped you think about what it means to be a woman? Where does menopause fit into the scheme of things?

6

Destination:
KEEPING PERSPECTIVE
ON YOUR HEALTH

JULIE

For over sixteen months, my whole view of my world and my health has changed. A close friend developed breast cancer, and although it was caught and dealt with, it was a chilling experience for everyone in our circle. The years of abuse another friend had put her body through, with poor diet, generally poor health habits, overworking, and excessive smoking, caught up with her, and she was dealing with one health problem or another most of the time. Then a coworker had a hysterectomy and was out of work for almost four weeks recovering. And during all this, my own body was starting to feel quite different.

I stopped having my period. Although I didn't miss it, I did miss the regularity and certainty of a monthly cycle, and I started wondering about my own health, especially considering what was going on with my friends. I started feeling a lot of aches and pains, and of course hot flashes and night sweats, and I was tired a lot. On top of that, everywhere I looked there was something cropping up about menopause. I figured I shouldn't just wait until maybe I discovered something unpleasant, so I started to read up on menopause and

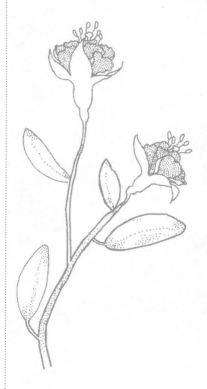

made an appointment to see my gynecologist. I feel like I'm being far more proactive now in thinking about and taking care of my health. It's just not something I take for granted anymore.

FOR MANY WOMEN, the passing into menopause may represent the first time that they've considered their health in the context of the *rest* of their lives. This alone signifies a major shift in thinking. Health care decisions now, which may begin to represent overall lifestyle decisions, have a *forward* thrust. How will these decisions affect you right now, *and* ten and twenty years into your future? What will health care choices today mean for your health tomorrow? Today's health care decisions are for you, and you alone. If you haven't had health care that's felt right for you, now is a good time to take the opportunity to think about and discover what feels good for you now and for your future.

Choosing care that's right for you pulls together a lot of different ideas, some of which have already been covered in earlier chapters. These include your approach to decision making, your preferences for traditional or alternative remedies, and the degree to which you throw yourself into learning about menopause and ways to deal with and treat it. However you are approaching menopause and gaining insight into this important life passage, taking the time to find care you can count on rather than just settling for what's familiar and already in place is an important step in taking control of your life. This chapter will help focus you on your health and the development of a health care plan for *life*.

Factors Affecting Health and Well-Being

We are complex biopsychosocial beings. We're more than just our physical being, our emotional and mental makeup, and our social relationships and interactions. And our health and our ability to be healthy is about more than just our physical well-being. The

World Health Organization has described health as "a state of complete physical, mental and social well-being, and not merely the absence of disease or infirmity."

Health, then, is healthy body *and* healthy mind. And we pretty much know that one affects the other. It's a popular belief that stress increases the chances of getting headaches and upset stomachs, and emotional tension is certainly related to heart disease. Likewise, lack of sleep or proper nutrition can have a profound effect on mood and emotions. Memory and concentration, for instance, are connected to both mood and physical health.

Accordingly, any problem that you encounter as you approach, enter, and pass through menopause may be influenced by many factors and result from multiple causes in your life. For instance, as discussed in Chapter 2, many men have similar experiences to women during the middle and later phases of their lives, including memory impairment, depression, weight gain, changes in emotional functioning and social relationships, and "midlife" crises. But they're definitely *not* experiencing menopause.

In fact, there are many things apart from menopause that can contribute to physical or emotional health problems during these middle years. Although the process of menopause can last many years from beginning to end, many women experience few or none of the major symptoms of menopause, and for many more women the signs and symptoms of menopause pass in a matter of months or a year or almost immediately with HRT. Despite this, however, women can still face significant changes in their physical and emotional health and well-being. For example, although depression in women has long been associated with menopause, many studies do not support this idea at all but instead just the opposite: depression in middle-age women is associated more with life circumstances, specific events and situations, relationships, and self-image than with menopause, as is the case with men who become depressed in their middle years. The reality is that

Our health and our ability to be healthy is about more than just our physical well-being. Health is healthy body and healthy mind.

many midlife issues are related more to this time in our development as *people* than to menopause.

Step back for a moment, and think about the things that might be contributing to physical or emotional health problems or concerns at this time in your life—things apart from the physical changes introduced by menopause and the aging process. Use the following journal entry to help focus your attention on what other factors in your life you should consider as you think about your health and plan for a lifetime health care strategy. Like most journal entries, this one provides a focal point and structure for your thinking, a way to get your own self-reflective juices flowing. Always use the checklists as a jumping off point, and take it from there, applying your own ideas and experiences to your writing.

Always use the checklists as a jumping-off point, and take it from there, applying your own ideas and experiences to your writing.

YOUR HEALTH ENVIRONMENT

1. What are some life factors besides your age and your menopause that might be contributing to changes in physical and emotional health and functioning? Check off any variable that in some way affects or risks your health, and add others that seem significant.

___*family history* (e.g., breast cancer in other family members, congenital conditions, and other medical issues that place you at risk through genetics)

___*nutrition and diet* (e.g., what you do and don't eat, when you eat, and how you eat)

___*physical condition* (e.g., being out of shape, not taking care of your body)

___*preexisting emotional problems* (e.g., poor mood, mood swings, low self-confidence and self-esteem, inability to manage feelings that predate perimenopause)

___*preexisting medical problems* (e.g., health and medical issues that predate perimenopause)

___*relationships* (e.g., relationships that are problematic, drain you, place demands that you have trouble meeting, or bother you in some significant manner) ___*sleep* (e.g., patterns of insomnia or restlessness, awakening midsleep, or oversleeping)

___*stress* (e.g., tensions from life, work, family, finances, expectations, and other responsibilities)

___*substance abuse* (e.g., excessive or routine use of alcohol or drugs that are taxing your ability to remain emotionally, mentally, or physically healthy)

___*toxins to the body* (e.g., tobacco, alcohol, caffeine, and other substances and foods that can poison your body through prolonged use)

___*worry* (e.g., concerns over relationships, finances, health, other people, job)

other: _____

_____

_____

2. Pick only one of the factors you checked off to serve as the focal point for the remainder of this entry, and explain why have you chosen this factor.

_____

_____

_____

3. Describe in what ways this factor does, or might, affect your health.

_____

_____

_____

_____

_____

4. What most concerns you about this risk factor to your health?

_____

_____

_____

_____

5. Is this an area of your life over which you can take some control, or is it outside your control?

_____

_____

_____

_____

6. Regardless of whether it is in or out of your direct control, can you exercise *some* control over this health risk factor?

_____

_____

_____

_____

7. What can you do to most affect this potential risk factor?

_____

_____

_____

_____

8. What will most likely stop you from taking whatever control you can?

_____

_____

_____

_____

_____

Your Personal Health

As you make assessments about your health and the many choices available to you to help with health and medical issues, it will be important to create a personal health inventory. Such an inventory will allow you to look back at your general health history, think about current risk factors, and make you more informed if you do seek out medical and health advice. In addition, a complete health inventory will include a review of family health history, something that most medical practitioners will want to know. A health inventory also acts as an ongoing resource for you because no one can remember all their important health details at any one time (nor do many people always realize the relevance of certain pieces of information that may take on different meanings when viewed as part of an overall health record).

A complete inventory should review and contain information about your family's history as well as your own, because it's important to know if certain types of medical or health problems have appeared among your immediate or extended family members or have recurred across generations of your family. In addition, a health inventory should gather information about your physical and mental health. It's particularly important to under-

A personal health inventory . . . will allow you both to look back at your general health history, think about current risk factors, and make you more informed should you decide to seek out medical and health advice.

stand your past physical and emotional responses and reactions if you're to make sense of your reactions in the present. A comprehensive inventory should contain information about:

- *Family history.* Include history of significant illnesses, diseases, or medical conditions or complications in parents, siblings, grandparents, and other members in your immediate family, with special focus on family history that may suggest certain medical treatments are contraindicated (i.e., clearly not recommended; family history of breast cancer, for instance, is a definite health risk in general and a risk for hormone therapies).

- *Mother's history of menopause.* Include age of menopause if known and mother's experience with menopause.

- *History of your menstrual periods.* Include age at onset, date of your last period, normal experience with and frequency of periods, your physical experiences and symptoms, and your mental and emotional experiences around the time of your periods.

- *Current physical health.* Include your estimate of your overall current health.

- *Current personal physical health conditions.* Include significant current conditions such as diabetes, asthma, fibroids, and allergies. As you learn more about hormone replacement therapy (HRT), you'll find that some diseases suggest HRT is contraindicated (e.g., current or a history of cancer presents a definite risk factor for use of estrogen therapies).

- *Physical health history.* Include a history of illnesses with emphasis on personal illnesses that suggest HRT is contraindicated.

- *Current physical condition.* Your self-assessment should address these questions: Are you in good shape? Do you work out?

Can you tolerate exercise? Are you underweight or over-weight?

- *Routine or recent medical tests or evaluations.* Include pap smears, mammograms, CAT or MRI scans, bone-density scan, saliva tests for hormone levels, cholesterol, ultrasound, and so on.

- *Current or recent indicators of menopause.* Include any signs such as hot flashes, night sweats, fatigue, and so on. (You may wish to review Chapter 2.)

- *History of pregnancy.* Include dates of and ages at pregnancies, childbirth, abortions, miscarriages, as well as physical and emotional experiences before, during, and after pregnancies.

- *Current mental, emotional, and cognitive health.* Include current mental health problems such as depression, anxiety, or other mood or emotional difficulties, problems with concentration or memory, or other current emotional or cognitive problems.

- *Mental health history.* Include history of prior mental health problems or difficulties and history of treatment, including past therapy or use of medications or herbal supplements.

- *Current medications, vitamins, and health or herbal supplements.* Include information about any medications, for both physical and emotional conditions, steroids, birth control, fertility drugs, and other supplements and treatments such as herbal, mineral, and vitamin, and how the medication is taken (e.g., orally, by patch, by injection, etc.).

- *Current health habits.* Include smoking or other use of tobacco, alcohol and drug use, caffeine consumption, and other habits related to diet and nutrition.

- *Current life stresses.* Although currently not part of most health inventories, understanding what stressors are active in your life is important as things like divorce, job loss, the death of someone close, or financial strain can significantly contribute to physical and mental illness.

* *Support network.* Having a support network is currently not an aspect of most health inventories, but having the support and assistance of family and friends, ministers, health care practitioners, and counselors can contribute a great deal to well-being, just as the absence of adequate support can be a significant threat to good health.

Take some time now to think about your health inventory, and complete at least a basic inventory. Then complete the following journal entry. (If you'd prefer, stop work altogether in your journal for now, and create a thorough inventory; then come back to this next entry when you're ready.)

YOUR HEALTH INVENTORY

1. What have you learned about your health history?

_____

_____

_____

_____

_____

2. Do you need to complete a more thorough personal inventory, or are you satisfied with the one you have?

_____

_____

_____

_____

3. Are there areas of your inventory that you need or want to work on in more detail or to research more?

_____

_____

_____

_____

_____

4. Does anything about your inventory startle or alarm you?

_____

_____

_____

_____

_____

5. Are there significant stresses in your life that are affecting your health or that might if not addressed and resolved soon?

_____

_____

_____

_____

_____

6. Do you have an adequate support system in place that meets your needs and is available to you as needed? If so, are you satisfied with the support available?

_____

_____

_____

_____

_____

7. How can you best use your health inventory to maintain or improve on your health as you move into your future?

_____

_____

_____

_____

8. Are there particular areas of your health or health assessment that you ought to follow up on?

_____

_____

_____

_____

THINGS TO THINK ABOUT

- Is it important to have a personal health inventory? If so, have you worked hard enough on developing your own?
- Are there health care issues that are of special concern to you? How will you follow up on these? Do you know where to get help?
- Have you been reading other books or materials on health and health-related issues? Should you be? Do you have all the medical and health information you need?

Taking Responsibility for Your Health

Although it's difficult to say exactly what you should be doing for your physical, mental, and spiritual health, we can say with relative certainty that the following ten guidelines will help you to stay healthy:

1. Don't smoke.

2. Limit your use of alcohol.

3. Limit your salt intake.

4. Limit and monitor your intake of saturated fats and cholesterol.

5. Eat adequate amounts of fiber, fruits, and vegetables.

6. Watch your diet for other excesses that may be unhealthy in large quantities.

7. Keep your body weight within the normal limits for your height, build, and age.

8. Get regular exercise, four to five times weekly.

9. Find ways to relax and reduce stress.

10. Remain active with friends and in the community.

These ten guidelines come together to define wellness as a combination of different types of healthy activities. Taking care of yourself in this way not only helps invigorate you but also fosters your ability to stay on top of things and think clearly. Use the next journal entry to examine your health and health practices.

A MAP FOR HEALTH

Think about each of the ten health areas cited above. They reflect basic tasks in remaining physically, emotionally, and spiritually healthy.

1. Think about how well you manage each area, and use the scale below to rate yourself. A score of 1 indicates that this area is not a health concern for you at all (e.g., perhaps you're not and have never been a smoker) or that you're well on top of the health issue (e.g., perhaps you used to smoke but have since quit). A score of 4 means that you either engage in clearly unhealthy behaviors (e.g., you eat a lot of foods heavy in fat

or drink alcohol heavily) or that you never think about your health practices in this particular area (e.g., you don't pay any attention to what you eat, or simply drink as much as you want whenever you want, without giving it a second thought).

Ten Healthy Practices	This is not a problem.	I watch this carefully.	I try but not too hard.	I pay no attention to this at all.
Don't smoke	1	2	3	4
Limit use of alcohol	1	2	3	4
Limit salt intake	1	2	3	4
Limit saturated fats/ cholesterol	1	2	3	4
Eat adequate fiber/ fruits/vegetables	1	2	3	4
Avoid excesses of unhealthy foods	1	2	3	4
Keep body weight within limits	1	2	3	4
Exercise regularly, 4–5 times weekly	1	2	3	4
Relax and reduce stress	1	2	3	4
Stay active with friends and community	1	2	3	4

2. Reviewing your answers to Question 1, are there any areas of your health practices that require some attention?

_____

_____

_____

_____

_____

3. If you see health problems or concerns, do they tend to fall in all three areas of body, mind, and spirit or in just one or two?

_____

_____

_____

_____

4. What can you do to improve your health in any or all three areas of wellness?

_____

_____

_____

_____

_____

_____

5. What *will* you do to maintain or improve your health?

_____

_____

_____

_____

_____

_____

THINGS TO THINK ABOUT

- Do you ever think of your physical or emotional health as a problem or concern? Even if you don't, are there other people in your life who express concern about your health?

- Do you take care of your body, or do you neglect it? Are you satisfied with your overall health, or should you be considering making a change in the way you think about your health?

Three Paths

There are three general pathways to take through your menopause. One involves changes in your lifestyle. This includes changes in diet, vitamin and mineral supplements, exercise and physical activity, individual therapy, support groups, and finding ways to reduce and manage stress through mind-body techniques (e.g., biofeedback, massage therapy, and yoga). For the most part, the intervention in these cases involves a change from *within*. A second pathway involves traditional medical interventions, usually in the form of HRT. The third pathway involves alternative medicine, and may include herbal remedies, eastern medicine, acupuncture and acupressure, and naturopathy. Like the traditional approach to medicine, here the focus is also on outside interventions, that is, something applied to the body to provide relief, bring about change, or alleviate a symptom.

Hormonal change is the primary reason that your body is experiencing the physical signs of menopause.

These three approaches, of course, can overlap. For instance, activities like yoga or meditation could be considered a lifestyle path or an alternative intervention. Many people choose interventions from all three categories, so know that you are not limited to any one area.

The Unavoidable Question of Hormone Replacement Therapy

You'll discover, if you haven't already, that no matter where you are on the perimenopause-menopause continuum, and no matter how you consider dealing with whatever troubles you, you'll be faced with the prospect of HRT.

Hormonal change is the primary reason that your body is experiencing the physical signs of menopause. In fact, the best and most acceptable reason for recommending and prescribing HRT is because it stems, and even reverses, many of the effects on the body that result from increasingly fluctuating and eventually diminishing hormone levels. For instance, estrogen is the hormone most typically associated with and responsible for female sexual characteristics, turning girls into women at puberty. It is a powerful hormone, and most of the body's cells have estrogen receptors on their surface. For this reason, estrogen influences hundreds of bodily processes, including the elasticity of blood vessels and skin, vaginal lubrication and strength, memory, bone density, and perhaps mood. As estrogen levels in the body decrease, the way your body functions, feels, behaves, and, in some cases, looks, changes as well. The same is true as well of other hormones that are being depleted, especially progesterone, the "other" hormone most associated with being female, producing your period and changing how you experience your body. In fact, your body *is* changing, and it is these changes that produce the physical "symptoms" of menopause, which in turn affect and shape the emotional and spiritual reality of the change. HRT can change this entire process by reintroducing the estrogen, progesterone, and/or testosterone that perimenopause takes away. That is why HRT has an effect on so many of the symptoms of menopause.

At its best, HRT is traditional medicine's response to the concerns of women. It replaces what menopause takes away—the steady and relatively predictable supply of the hormones. In doing so, HRT changes the course and impact of menopause on the body, mind, and spirit. Along with the risks it may bring, HRT can reverse many of the symptoms and signs of menopause and correct physical problems that may be developing. For many women, HRT brings both physical and emotional relief and can quickly change the menopausal experience.

The *least* acceptable and most suspect reason for seeing hormone replacement so widely advertised, recommended, and prescribed is because of its commercial value. With unprecedented numbers of women currently entering menopause, HRT means

Estrogen influences hundreds of bodily processes, including the elasticity of blood vessels and skin, vaginal lubrication and strength, memory, bone density, and perhaps mood.

There are medical risks to the introduction of hormones into the body, some of which are well documented.

big money for the pharmaceutical companies who produce and sell it, and there's always the risk of overselling or overprescribing a product for commercial (and not necessarily medically legitimate) reasons. In addition, the entire HRT approach leads to what some have termed the "medicalization" of menopause. Some people believe that they have a "deficiency disease" that needs to be "fixed" by hormone replacement. The message they've heard is that they'll be old before their time if they don't receive HRT. For many, aside from the issues and concerns about the long-term use of a hormone replacement in the body, the idea that they *have* to take a hormone replacement to deal with a natural process is objectionable and suggests that women can't live a successful, satisfying, and medically healthy life any other way.

Commercialism and philosophy aside, there are medical risks to the introduction of hormones into the body, some of which are well documented. Women with a history of cancer or diabetes in themselves or their family, for instance, are often advised not to take an estrogen supplement (the issues are less clear regarding HRT for women with diabetes, but precaution and discussion is still urged), and estrogen is frequently not recommended for women who have experienced heart disease. Also, there are side effects and risks associated with HRT, many of which are not fully known or understood at this time.

The most usual hormonal regimen is a combination of estrogen and progesterone. At present, there's considerable controversy about including testosterone in this regimen as well (for the purpose of increasing sexual desire). HRT can take several forms from pills to patches, and new ideas about dosage are being presented as new data are analyzed.

Not every women will need a hormone replacement therapy. Some women continue to produce enough hormones after their menopause to suffice, minimizing physical changes. And hormones are stored and metabolized in fatty tissue, so some women will have more hormones in "storage" than others (for once, it might be an advantage to have a little extra fat!). The level of hormones produced by the adrenal glands and the amount stored in fatty tissues varies from woman to woman, which is another reason why a decision on hormonal replacement is both a very individual matter *and* one that needs to be revisited regularly. Starting HRT, for example, does not mean remaining on HRT for the rest of your life, although it may for some women.

There are dozens of facts and ideas to be learned about HRT and the various forms and combinations in which it is prescribed and administered. You can read about these in any number of excellent books that focus on menopause, and you can keep up to date through magazine articles, news shows, and the Internet. Regardless of whether you choose to do this research yourself, stay in touch with your trusted health care practitioner. She or he can help you to decide whether you need or can be helped by HRT for any problems you may be encountering as you pass through menopause. If you don't have a health practitioner you feel comfortable with or fully trust, it's a good idea to start looking for one.

The Alternatives

Many women do not feel compelled to pursue any interventions at all for their menopause. Whatever signs and symptoms they may experience never rise to the point where they are intrusive or difficult to deal with. Other women, however, do seek assistance or relief from the effects of menopause, and for different reasons. Many choose to not go the HRT route.

There are numerous alternatives to HRT that range from dietary and vitamin regimens to herbal remedies, homeopathy, acupuncture, acupressure, and meditation. There are more alter-

There are numerous alternatives to HRT that range from dietary and vitamin regimens to herbal remedies, homeopathy, acupuncture, acupressure, and meditation.

natives than can be easily listed here, but once again there exists a plethora of fine books, support groups, women's centers, and other resources that can inform and instruct you about these many alternatives.

Millions of people use, count on, and swear by alternatives of every kind. Some alternatives will probably cause no harm even if they fail to fix the problem (such as vitamin or mineral supplements); others will prove to be useful regardless of their ability to solve problems associated with menopause (such as psychotherapy, meditation, biofeedback, and physical exercise). Regardless of their impact on menopause, the lifestyle alternatives are the most likely to help your spirit and emotions and possibly get you physically fit and healthy at the same time. Time honored herbal remedies, even if they fail to produce a change in your menopausal symptoms, may well give you a sense of self-control, direction, and focus that will be useful.

Use this next journal entry to think about the three paths through menopause and to sort out your thinking about interventions and menopause.

WHICH PATH?

1. What sort of approaches to menopause do you consider to be lifestyle oriented?

_____

_____

_____

2. Which lifestyle interventions do you most favor using?

_____

_____

_____

_____

3. Are you interested in any of the "alternative" approaches to medicine? If so, which aspects or interventions?

_____

_____

_____

_____

4. Do you need to learn more about alternative medical approaches?

_____

_____

_____

5. Does the traditional medical approach feel most right, least right, or somewhere in between for you?

_____

_____

_____

_____

6. How does the traditional medical approach to menopause fit with your experience and needs at this time?

_____

_____

_____

_____

7. Are you at a point where you're even ready to think about HRT or any other intervention?

_____

_____

_____

_____

8. Based on what you already know, is HRT a route you want to explore?

_____

_____

_____

9. If HRT is something you'd rather avoid, what alternatives are you considering? If HRT is an intervention you want to pursue, what do you need to know about it?

_____

_____

_____

_____

_____

THINGS TO THINK ABOUT

- Do you have a trusted medical practitioner you can turn to for advice and help? Do you have anyone else you can discuss your questions and thoughts with?
- Have you listened to the stories of other women who have tried different approaches to dealing with menopause? Have you turned to others who have walked this road ahead of you to learn from their experiences?
- Which path—traditional, alternative, or lifestyle—most resonates for you and most seems to fit your situation? Can you blend all three?

Major Risks to Women's Health

You may already know that heart disease, breast and colorectal cancer, and osteoporosis are considered major causes of death and disability in older women today. In fact, as you age, heart disease becomes the *number one* risk factor to your health, despite the frightening statistics and great deal of concern legitimately directed toward breast cancer. Although many people think of heart disease and heart failure as a "man's" illness, it is the leading cause of death for women over the age of 45. As you enter and pass through perimenopause and menopause, the changes in your body increase your risk of heart disease, in part due to a reduction in estrogen that affects the elasticity of veins and arteries as well as affecting cholesterol. Estrogen is believed to help keep the "good" cholesterol (HDL) up, while keeping "bad" cholesterol (LDL) down.

Osteoporosis is another major health risk for women. Once callously known as dowager's hump because it can deform the skeletal structure and lead to a hunched over and huddled posture, osteoporosis causes bone degeneration, brittle bones, curvature of the spine, and shrinkage of the skeleton, actually reducing height. This condition can also lead to other problems such as increased risk of bone fractures and other serious injuries. Many women over the age of 50 are at risk for this disease, and perhaps 25% of women will develop some version of this disease in their lifetime. Aptly known as the silent thief, there are few symptoms of osteoporosis until you break a bone, suffer joint damage, or feel the permanent effects of bone mass loss in aches and pains.

You are at risk for these diseases just because you're aging. The same is true for men as well as women, although the changing landscape of women's bodies as they pass through menopause certainly increases the risk. There are some risk factors you simply can't change.

- *Family factors.* A family history of a particular disease suggests that you may have some greater genetic predisposition to that illness or disease.

- *Race.* The risks for particular diseases vary from race to race: for instance, African American women experience higher rates of heart disease than Caucasian women, and Asian and Caucasian women suffer relatively higher rates of osteoporosis than African American and Hispanic women.

- *Other health conditions.* Diabetes if uncontrolled, for instance, has an effect on arteries throughout the body and doubles your chance of coronary disease.

The good news is that there are also health risks that you *can* influence and change. Some of these issues and ideas were addressed earlier in this chapter, and you already thought some about some of your health choices and behaviors ("A Map for Health" journal entry). Despite the risks, there are *many* things you can do to manage and take care of your health right now, as well as shape your future health.

- *Stop smoking.* Smoking increases your risk for cancer, high blood pressure, and heart disease, and it depletes calcium from your bones.

- *Start exercising.* Maintain your cardiovascular system and muscle tone.

- *Watch your diet and nutrition.* Ensure you're eating well-balanced meals that include the vitamin and mineral supplements recommended for menopause and the aging process in general.

- *Use alcohol only in moderation.* Alcohol can cause serious and significant health-threatening conditions as well as increase blood pressure and the risk of heart failure.

- *Ensure your weight is within the established range for your age, height, and build.* Being significantly over- *or* underweight robs your body of the nutrition it needs and increases your chances for heart failure or other major health problems.

- *Take care of other significant health risks or current health problems.*

Other health problems such as high blood pressure, diabetes, and high cholesterol leave you more susceptible to illness.

- *Reduce stress in your life.* It's no surprise that people under stress are more prone to illness than those who manage to cope effectively with stress.

- *Get routine physical exams.* An ounce of prevention is worth a pound of cure—pap smears, mammograms, cholesterol and lipid profiles, bone density scans, and other routine check-ups are an excellent way to spot problems *before* they begin.

Your Health Care Provider

The people who help you make informed decisions for yourself, or who you allow to make decisions for you, are enormously important in your life. There are many people, professions, and disciplines that purport to know a great deal about menopause. Remember, though, that there are many ways to approach this change of life, and many opinions may be more philosophical or sociological in nature than medical or health related. Remember too, however, that menopause is a physical event as well as life-changing passage, and it has potential medical and other health implications. For this reason, it is important to have a trusted medical practitioner.

Whether you see a family physician, a physician who specializes in women's health, a nurse practitioner, or some other health care provider, it's important to have someone on your side to whom you can turn for expert knowledge, someone who is informed about menopause research and practice and who is able to advise, prescribe, and practically help you through the medical and health implications of this change. Do you have such a person in your life?

Use this final journal entry to think about your medical advisor and health care provider, as well as your general health.

Menopause is a physical event as well as a life-changing passage, and it has potential medical and other health implications.

TO YOUR HEALTH

1. What are you willing to do to take care of your health?

_____

_____

_____

_____

2. Are there health changes you need to make? If so, are these lifestyle, medical, or attitude changes?

_____

_____

_____

_____

3. What do you seek in a health care provider? Check off the items that most fit, and below add other qualities that are important to you.

a. Gender of practitioner:

__female   __male   __doesn't matter

b. Health profession:

__traditional medical doctor   __nurse practitioner   __nontraditional medicine

other: _____

_____

c. Primary base of practice:

__alternative medicine   __holistic   __traditional medicine

__general health practice   __natural medicine   __women's health focus

other: _____

_____

_____

d. Primary approach to interventions:

__aggressive treatment of symptoms   __minimal interventions

__interventions used as last resort   __rapid response to symptoms

__least intrusive measures   __thorough evaluation before interventions

other: _____   _____

_____   _____

_____   _____

_____   _____

e. Primary attitude toward patients:

__assertive   __distant   __open   __supportive

__businesslike   __engaging   __opinioned   __take-control

__considerate   __laid back   __sharing   __warm

other: _____   _____

_____   _____

_____   _____

4. What do your answers to Question 3 tell you about your preferred health care practitioner?

_____

_____

_____

_____

_____

5. What do these answers tell you about your health care needs?

_____

_____

_____

6. Do you have a medical practitioner or health care provider you really trust?

_____

_____

_____

_____

_____

THINGS TO THINK ABOUT

- Do you need to spend more time focusing on your health care issues and needs?
- Are you satisfied with your primary health care provider?
- Have you asked other women about their experiences with health providers?

7

Destination:
EMOTIONS AND MOODS

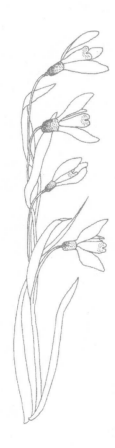

LOUISE

My husband wondered what was wrong. He felt that my emotions were off track, and said it reminded him of when I got pregnant. He felt he had to watch every word he said, and was never sure how I was going to react. I was defensive at first—actually, I was furious. I felt he didn't understand me at all. It was only after he agreed that he didn't understand me recently, and said he couldn't understand why I was so angry with him, that I started to think maybe he had a point. I was so caught up in my emotions that I hadn't even noticed just how moody I'd become. I made an appointment with my doctor, and it became clear that I was menopausal. Soon after, I started HRT and I found my emotional self returning to normal.

MARKIE

I expected my emotions to go through the wall when I entered menopause. But they never did. I definitely experienced some big changes in how my body seemed to be working and felt a lot of physical changes. That raised some anxiety for me, but I never really hit that emotional wall that I'd heard about. Still, it was useful for me to be aware of possible emotional changes, because it kept me alert and kept me very tuned into myself. I've never been an especially emotional person, but I'm certainly far more aware of my emotions now than before my menopause.

CERTAIN PARTS OF the brain are larger in women than in men. These areas are more active during emotional interactions and are considered especially sensitive to emotional influences and experiences. For this reason, many argue that a woman's brain is designed to be tuned in and responsive to mood and emotion.

Menopause does not cause depression.

Moods do shift during menopause for many reasons, but there is no reason to believe that depression itself has much to do with menopause. In fact, as a group, women in their fifties have the lowest rates of depression compared with women at any other stage of life. Furthermore, clinical depression is rare among menopausal women. Studies show that perimenopausal women experiencing depression were often women who had experienced depression during their premenopausal years, and women who are especially emotional during menopause are likely to be women who were especially emotional in their premenopausal years.

Menopause does not *cause* depression. Actually, menopausal women who are experiencing mood swings, depression, and anxiety are likely to have other events going on in their lives that are contributing to these emotional shifts and episodes. This is not to say that hormonal fluctuations and changes don't affect mood. They do, and this is true for all people. However, while our bodies may be influenced by hormonal changes, severe emotional problems are more likely related to personality, psychological makeup, and real-life events rather than simply a changing physiology.

Emotions play a prominent part in the lives of all people, and this is no less true of women passing through menopause. Why would it be? Just as for men, entering midlife is a time of many changes and personal questions for women too. During these years much changes, from our bodies and health to families that are growing up, illness and death among our own parents and peers, and a sense of our own mortality. On top of that, women *are* going through very real physical changes, and, until the last few years, they had been flooded with the idea that the loss of their childbearing years signaled a loss of their overall purpose and vitality too. Add to that the images presented to us all by the mass media of "beautiful," "attractive," and "sexy" women, most of whom are young and groomed by the media, and it's no wonder that many women feel emotionally fragile, unsure of themselves, and even panicked at times. But these are not the "symptoms" of menopause; they are the products of a society that has, until recently, defined and ascribed value to women based on their age and physical attractiveness to men.

Just as for men, entering midlife is a time of many changes and personal questions for women too.

In this chapter, you'll have the chance to think about the *normal* emotions experienced by most people and some of the experiences and emotions that may be especially tied to this change in your life. The goals of this chapter are to help you recognize the normalcy of moods and emotions, understand the basis of your emotions, and find ways to both recognize and regulate your emotions so that they assist your personal growth rather than impede it.

Feelings

No one really knows completely how our minds work or how we experience, make sense of, and respond to the world. Some consider feelings to be the "shadows" and products of our thoughts. Others see feelings as more primitive and basic than thought—an instinctual response to the world around us. By still others, feelings and thoughts are considered just another type of behavior and response to our environment. Whatever their origin, feelings describe your often *immediate* response to your world and the things that make up that world. Although many people don't know how to explain or can't find the words to describe their feelings, most people know exactly what feelings are because they experience them directly.

Not every feeling is a good one. People experience both negative and positive feelings. Many people go through a period when their predominant feelings are negative and difficult to manage. Sometimes these negative feelings are the direct result of a specific situation or event, such as a death or a divorce. At other times, they may feel unattached to anything in particular; they just feel "bad." The same can be said of the positive feelings. Sometimes people feel on top of the world because something good has happened; at other times, they just feel good for no particular reason.

No matter what the feeling, or where it comes from, it is an important guide. Feelings point to your experience of the world in the moment. Even though you might tell yourself (or others might tell you) you should feel okay, your own feelings usually prevail. Most people can't easily shake off a bad feeling or get talked out of a bad mood. However, even though some feelings are difficult to accept or deal with, it's not the goal of any kind of reflective work to find ways to eliminate or bypass unpleasant feelings. Instead, the purpose is to find ways to recognize and accept difficult feelings and learn to tolerate, manage, and work through them. Feelings, even bad ones, can help you gauge what's right for you and what's wrong. If you're in touch with your feelings, not just trying to get rid of the negative ones, they can help point to the issues that are affecting you and provide direction in how best to deal with these triggers. Unfortunately, some people can't recognize their own feelings or are only able to recognize their most familiar emotions.

Feelings describe your often immediate *response to your world and the things that make up that world.*

Factors Influencing Your Feelings

During the years leading up to menopause, your moods and emotions may have varied considerably. In many ways, how you deal with and feel about menopause will be determined by who you are and what you bring to this time in your life, rather than menopause itself. In fact, it's important to realize that although menopause may introduce significant life changes and new ideas, it does *not* bring about severe emotional instability or change. Nevertheless, the changes and stresses of menopause may combine with other life issues and your emotional coping style to put you in touch with a series of feelings, some of which may be difficult to deal with. This serves as an advantage in that you may now be able to deal with issues that might otherwise have remained under the surface for years to come. A variety of factors may influence your feelings as you enter and deal with the issues in your life at this time.

Even though some feelings are difficult to accept or deal with, it is not the goal of any kind of reflective work to find ways to eliminate or bypass unpleasant feelings.

- *Your knowledge about what you're experiencing.* The more you can educate yourself about your physical, emotional, and spiritual changes and what they mean for your future, the better prepared you'll be to deal with feelings that may spring up unexpectedly, and the better able you'll be to distinguish between different kinds of feelings and their sources.

- *Your general state of health.* If you're basically healthy, the chances are that you'll be able to withstand a variety of stressors. If you have significant health problems, the usual physical and emotional stresses of menopause may be more problematic. (You may want to review Chapter 6.)

- *The physical impact of menopause.* If you pass through these menopausal years with minor signs of change and little difficulty, or if you have decided to begin early hormone replacement therapy, your moods may be little affected by fluctuating hormones. On the other hand, if you've had wildly fluctuating hormonal levels, with accompanying hot flashes, sleep loss, aching bones, and other menopausal signs, myriad feelings may be evoked due to hormonal changes, physical stress, and your response to your experience. Add to this the fact that estrogen (one of those major hormones that's fluctuating during menopause and on the wane after) also enhances serotonin, a natural chemical transmitter in the body that has a positive effect on one's sense of well-being, then, it is easy to see that a decrease in estrogen may also have an impact on mood.

If your relationships are comfortable and supportive, chances are they will help you to deal with and withstand new developments in your life.

- *The quality and overall state of your relationships.* If your relationships are comfortable and supportive, chances are they will help you to deal with and withstand new developments in your life. On the other hand, if you're in a conflict about an important relationship, or your relationships are generally unfulfilling, the combination of relationship problems and menopause may lead to intense feelings that "bubble" to the surface from where they may once have been suppressed.

- *The amount of "unfinished" business in your life.* If there are important issues you haven't dealt with in your life, they may come to the surface now. If you've been avoiding decisions about relationships, career, education, or health, or if there are significant issues from an earlier time in your life left unaddressed or unresolved, they too may surface. Like other emotions that arise during this time, the emergence of these issues can also lead to great gains.

- *The type and amount of stress in your life.* Everyone deals with stress in a different way. Where some may thrive, others may crumble. Menopause can, undoubtedly, combine with other stressful aspects of your life to become part of a highly charged emotional environment.

- *Your prior experience with mood swings, emotional difficulties, depression, anxiety, and other significant emotional or mental health problems.* If you have a history of strong emotional responses, difficulties dealing with emotional situations, or mental health issues, you may be more susceptible during and after menopause to strong and unsettling emotional reactions. The opposite is equally true. If you've always been able to easily or appropriately handle emotions and use them to your advantage, this history is likely to accompany you through this current passage in your life.

- *Your history with past losses, life stressors, and change.* Your previous experiences with loss and change will influence your emotional responses during this time in your life. If menopause comes after a series of losses or major changes, or you experience menopause as one more loss in your life, it's more likely to have a negative impact on your emotions. And the way you've dealt with loss and change in the past will have a bearing. Even "good" changes, such as a new relationship or a new job, can contribute to emotional stress if too many changes are taking place at the same time.

- *Your sense of who you are and who you want to be.* As menopause is typically a midlife event, here's where those potential midlife issues may come into play. You are faced with some inescapable evidence of aging. Ideas about who you are, who you want to be, and how you view the rest of your life are all important factors in your emotional well-being and can affect your ability to deal with the issues that may be involved in menopause.

If menopause comes after a series of losses or major changes, or you experience menopause as one more loss in your life, it's likely to have a negative impact on your emotions.

It's not that any one of these factors alone will explain your emotional condition at this point in your life or predict your emotional future. Most important is an analysis of *your* personal life factors, which, acting together, will influence your moods and your emotions.

You may wish to reassess your emotional condition and connect it to the six attributes of wellness described in Chapter 3: self-acceptance, purpose, environmental mastery, personal growth, positive relationships, and autonomy.

Becoming Aware of Feelings

Before you can express a feeling, you have to first realize you're *having* one. And to prevent yourself from being swept away by a powerful feeling, you must first think about and understand it. Recognizing that you have a feeling is the bridge that connects your thoughts to your emotions. In fact, almost everything you do in this journal is a product of your thinking about your feelings and your experiences in general. Expression refers to venting and managing your emotions in a way that supports self-knowledge and personal growth. Of course, writing about feelings isn't the only way to express them. In fact, people quite frequently vent their feelings without any thought at all.

Acting out happens when there's no conscious connection between feelings and behaviors; the term is usually used when someone inappropriately acts out a feeling of some kind, without thought.

"Acting out" happens when there's no conscious connection between feelings and behaviors; the term is usually used when someone inappropriately "acts out" a feeling of some kind, without thought. But there are many times when it's important to behave spontaneously, without thinking about it. Crying, for instance, is an example of spontaneous behavior that is often a very appropriate way to let off emotional energy. On the other hand, yelling at someone because you're angry is not a particularly positive way to let off steam, nor is overeating or drinking too much alcohol. These are examples of acting out an emotion in a way that may be destructive to your relationships and yourself. As you work through this time of change in your life, one goal is to express your feelings in ways that are positive, healthy, and contribute to personal growth. Critical to this goal is your ability to recognize and understand your feelings. This process is a step toward emotional *regulation*. Regulation doesn't stop your feelings; it helps you express them positively, instead of acting them out. Simply put, coping with a feeling doesn't mean you don't have them. But it does mean you don't let them overwhelm you. Something as simple as stopping to think about how you're feeling at a difficult moment can be a useful way to regulate and cope with that emotion.

The next journal entry will help you recognize how you're feeling, and why. It provides a checklist of basic feelings, some of which you may experience during this time in your life. Complete the entry shortly before or after experiencing a situation that may be emotional for you or when you find feelings washing over you. It's a simple way to help pick up on and understand a feeling.

MY FEELINGS

How I Feel   **Why I Feel This Way**

___abandoned   _____

___afraid   _____

___angry   _____

___anxious   _____

___ashamed   _____

___bitter   _____

___dejected   _____

___detached   _____

__disappointed   _____

__disregarded   _____

__foolish   _____

__guilty   _____

__happy   _____

__helpless   _____

__hopeful   _____

__hopeless   _____

__ignored   _____

__incapable   _____

__irritated   _____

__lonely   _____

__numb   _____

__overwhelmed   _____

__sad   _____

__trapped   _____

__vulnerable   _____

__worthless   _____

THINGS TO THINK ABOUT

- Were you easily able to pick out feelings? If you've used this journal format more than once, is it getting easier to recognize your feelings?
- Do you understand why you feel the way you do? Is it important to understand how you feel?
- Do you want to be able to regulate your feelings? Does understanding your feelings help you to regulate them?

Understanding Your Feelings

To understand your feelings, you have to go beyond simple recognition. *Interoceptive* awareness is the ability to correctly recognize and interpret feelings as you have them. It is about knowing *how* you feel. People with poor interoceptive awareness often misidentify their feelings. *Introspective* awareness, on the other hand, is understanding *why* you feel the way you do. Introspection is looking "inside"—focusing in on your own thoughts and feelings. Sometimes people find it difficult to look at themselves in this way, but taking the time to think about your feelings and reflect on your thoughts is one way to better know yourself and adjust to the world around you. By linking your feelings to your thoughts, you also link your feelings to your behaviors. You stop behaving impulsively or reactively. You begin to see yourself more clearly and understand why and how you respond to things, including this change in your life. In turn, you're better able to see *how* to respond and what actions to take.

The next journal entry will help you zero in on individual feelings and provide structure to start to understand them.

> Interoceptive *awareness is the ability to correctly recognize and interpret feelings as you have them.*

THINKING ABOUT YOUR FEELINGS

1. Think about the previous journal entry. At this time in you life, which emotions are the most difficult for you to manage? Pick six for this entry.

a. _____   d. _____

b. _____   e. _____

c. _____   f. _____

2. Pick one of these emotions for this entry, and describe it in words.

_____

_____

_____

_____

3. Why is this feeling so difficult to handle?

_____

_____

_____

_____

_____

4. What situations or events seem to lead to this feeling?

_____

_____

_____

_____

5. How do you generally handle this feeling?

_____

_____

_____

_____

6. Are you satisfied with the way you handle the feeling?

_____

_____

_____

_____

7. What changes might you make to better handle this feeling in the future?

_____

_____

_____

_____

THINGS TO THINK ABOUT

- Have you learned more about this feeling? Was your feeling more complicated then you initially thought it was?
- If you've used this journal format more than once, are you learning more about your feelings? What are you learning?
- Does understanding your feelings help you manage them?

Your Changing Feelings

As you age and develop as a person, you change. This is also true of your emotions; that is, the quality, or "feel," of your emotions has probably changed as well. You're not the same person you were twenty or even ten years ago, and you're going through a powerful change in your life right now. It would be surprising, then, if you experienced emotions the same way now as you did when you were younger and less experienced.

As you know, in addition to the process of development and maturation, there are many factors that can shape or directly affect your emotions. One powerful factor, of course, is your changing body and, in particular, changing hormones. As a complicated being, your emotions are no less complicated. Nevertheless, a significant part of managing emotions so that they don't manage *you* is thinking about them and trying to make sense of their relationship to your larger life.

A significant part of managing emotions so that they don't manage you is thinking about them and trying to make sense of their relationship to your larger life.

Use the next journal entry to think about your current emotional condition in general. What's changed, what's difficult to deal with, and what can your emotions teach you about yourself? Like many of the journal entries, there are no correct answers, and there's no one right way to answer the questions. Although some journal entries in the book call for answers that are undeliberated and spontaneous, in this case think carefully about each question before answering it. Use the entry to really think about (and feel) emotional changes.

YOUR CHANGING FEELINGS

1. What has most changed about your emotions over the past few years, especially recently?

_____
_____
_____
_____

2. Do your emotions feel as though they're sometimes out of your control?

_____
_____
_____
_____

3. Do you express your emotions adequately?

_____
_____
_____
_____
_____

4. What most prevents you from expressing your emotions?

_____

_____

_____

_____

_____

5. What can most help you to express your emotions?

_____

_____

_____

_____

_____

6. What most confuses you about your emotions?

_____

_____

_____

_____

7. What most concerns you about your emotions?

_____

_____

_____

_____

8. Complete these sentences.

a. *Sometimes my emotions are like . . .* _____

b. *Sometimes, I just feel like I . . .* _____

c. *If I don't let my emotions out, I . . .* _____

d. *If I don't let my emotions out, they* . . . _____

e. *If I do let my emotions out* . . . _____

9. How are changing emotions a reflection of your changing self?

_____

_____

_____

_____

_____

Feelings and Moods

Some feelings last a while and are more like a collection of feelings, rather than a single emotion. Sometimes one feeling is so persistent and long lasting that it takes over how you see things or deal with situations. This is a *mood*, or a single underlying feeling or set of feelings that colors everything for you while in that mood.

Sometimes one feeling is so persistent and long lasting that it takes over how you see things or deal with situations. This is a mood.

There are good moods and bad ones—happy, angry, satisfied, depressed. Moods are only thought of as problems when they frequently fluctuate from high to low or when the most common mood is a bad mood of some kind. When moods are pervasive over time, they sometimes begin to interfere with your ability to function and with the quality of your life. At that point, a mood may be developing into a disorder that needs treatment. For instance, if you're often depressed and you find that *everything* is affected by your mood—your sleep, your appetite, your energy, your ability to concentrate—this may be a problem. The same is true if you're anxious all the time or angry. Moods can become so deep that they change the way you see and feel about everything.

As you move through your menopause, you'll no doubt experience many moods. Most of these you will overcome, but if others seem insurmountable you should consider discussing your moods with your health care practitioner.

The most useful time to write about a feeling is when you're having it, and the most useful time to think about a mood is when you're in it. Accordingly, complete the next journal entry only when you're in the grip of a mood. Look over the entry now, but skip it and return only when you can write about a mood you're actually experiencing. You may not *want* to write when in an emotionally difficult mood, but this is the challenge. It is designed to help you make sense of your life. Of course, not all moods are bad. Some moods are lighthearted and fun. All moods are important to write about, so don't limit your entries to only unpleasant or bad moods. Remember to think about your positive moods too.

All moods are important to write about, so don't limit your entries to unpleasant or bad moods.

HOW DO YOU FEEL RIGHT NOW

1. What kind of mood are you in?

_____

_____

_____

_____

2. Describe your mood in a single word. _____

3. What are the main emotions in this mood?

_____

_____

_____

_____

4. Put your mood into words by completing these sentences.

a. *This mood is . . .* _____

_____

_____

b. *If this mood had a color, it would be . . .* _____

c. *If this mood had texture, it would be . . .* _____

d. *If this mood made a sound, it would be . . .* _____

e. *If this mood had a scent, it would be . . .* _____

5. Describe your mood in words. *I feel . . .* _____

_____

_____

_____

_____

6. What brought this mood on?

_____

_____

_____

_____

7. How long have you been feeling this way?

_____

_____

8. Is this a common mood for you?

_____

_____

_____

9. Is this mood so strong that it's interfering with your daily life?

_____

_____

_____

_____

THINGS TO THINK ABOUT

- If this is an unpleasant mood, what can you do to avoid situations that contribute to this mood? If this is a pleasant mood, what sort of situations or relationships stimulate this mood and keep it alive?
- Have the types or frequency of your moods changed over time, and especially since entering perimenopause? In what ways?
- Are your moods so long lasting or intense that they affect your ability to function? If they are, do you feel you need help with them?

Dealing with Feelings

Knowing that you have feelings and being able to identify them are important steps in managing your emotions. But knowing you're angry or sad doesn't necessarily mean you know how to deal with the feeling. Dealing with a feeling means working it out in a way that both brings relief and is healthy and appropriate. Many people, however, behave in ways that are self-destructive or self-defeating in an attempt to eliminate a difficult feeling

Dealing with a feeling means working it out in a way that both brings relief and is healthy and appropriate.

rather than learning to deal with and work through it. These sorts of behaviors include excessive drinking, aggression, overeating or undereating, and other types of behavior that are self-harming, harmful to others, or antisocial. Their behaviors not only fail to help but actually serve to make problems worse. Essentially, dealing with feelings comes down to four steps:

1. *Tolerate the feeling.* This involves accepting it, putting up with it, and finding a way to live with it.

2. *Cope with the pressure of the feeling.* Find a way to ensure that the feeling doesn't push you into behavior that you know is bad for you, bad for others, or in some other way inappropriate. Find a way to let off the emotional steam in ways that aren't self-destructive or self-defeating.

3. *Listen to the feeling.* Understand the meaning of the emotion: why you're feeling this way, what might be causing the feeling, and what the feeling is "telling" you about the situation.

4. *Respond to the feeling.* Find an appropriate response to the feeling. Sometimes this means telling someone how you feel; sometimes it means being alone, and sometimes it means crying, yelling, or not doing anything at all.

Each one of these steps is important, and one leads to the next until the feeling has been processed and is no longer acting as a source of pressure. "Dealing" with a feeling means that you've expressed the emotional pressure and can move on without being controlled by the emotion. In the ideal emotional situation, dealing with a feeling involves all four of these steps, but each step is important in its own right. Even if you never get to the second step in this sequence, just tolerating the feeling has great value. Regardless of the intensity of your emotions, you must learn how to deal with them.

Coping Behaviors

Your behavior is your outward expression of what's going on inside of you. Although others can't see the inside of your mind or read your thoughts, they can see how you deal with this inner experience. Behavior includes the things you actually do, like yelling, crying, moping, getting angry, or laughing, as well as the things you say. It includes the things that people observe about you, such as your attitude, body language, and how you spend your time. Behavior also includes the things you don't do—for example not speaking to someone, not attending a meeting, or not finishing something you started. In other words, your behaviors include every facet of your interactions with the world and the people in it. Just as there's no such thing as *non*action, there's no such thing as *non*behavior.

There are many kinds of behaviors, including behavior that helps us to deal with feelings and situations. Coping behaviors are those things we do to help express and vent emotional pressure. They improve, not worsen, our situation and strengthen our ability to deal with issues. So-called negative coping behaviors are really *attempts* at coping that don't work. Effective coping, however, is always healthy and entails:

Negative coping behaviors are really attempts *at coping* that don't work.

- knowing when you have feelings—being in touch with what's going on inside

- identifying feelings—recognizing and being able to name the feelings

- tolerating feelings—accepting the feelings, and not trying to escape them

- managing feelings—controlling your feelings, not letting them control you

- understanding feelings—connecting your feelings to their causes
- expressing feelings—allowing your feelings to emerge and be expressed

Focus your next entry on your coping behaviors. Your writing will help you not only to think about ways to deal with your feelings but behaviors to avoid when you experience difficult emotions.

COPING BEHAVIORS

1. How do you deal with your feelings?

_____

_____

_____

_____

_____

2. Can you tolerate difficult feelings?

_____

_____

_____

_____

3. Do you give in to your feelings and act on them without thinking?

_____

_____

_____

_____

_____

4. Do you listen to your feelings and understand where they're coming from or what they're trying to tell you?

_____

_____

_____

_____

5. Do you respond appropriately to your feelings?

_____

_____

_____

_____

6. What's the healthiest way you deal with your feelings?

_____

_____

_____

_____

7. Do you ever get caught in, or create, self-defeating cycles of behavior that hinder or hurt you instead of helping to appropriately express feelings?

_____

_____

_____

_____

8. Are your behaviors and responses to your feelings ever self-destructive or self-defeating?

_____

_____

_____

_____

9. Which of your behaviors are the healthiest in dealing with your feelings?

_____

_____

_____

_____

THINGS TO THINK ABOUT

- Was it difficult to look at your behaviors? What did you learn about yourself?
- Is your behavioral style helping, hindering, or hurting you? Are there behavioral patterns you need to think more about or change?
- Do you ever hide your behaviors from others? If so, why?

Checkpoint: Thoughts on Your Menopause

Menopause is experienced differently by different women. The same sign of menopause may be seen by one woman as a symptom of a problem, by another as a signpost of a new stage in her life, and by a third as a temporary aberration. There is no "right" way to feel. There is only _your_ way. Recognizing the power of perspective, then, what are your thoughts now about this time in your life? Is this stage experienced mainly as a plus or a minus? The answers to questions like these will influence your feelings and moods during menopause and beyond.

8

Destination:

BIOGRAPHY

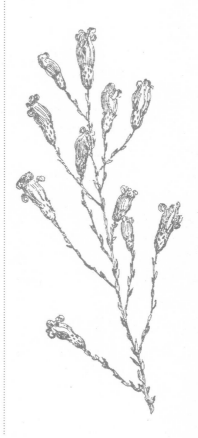

DAWN

When I first entered menopause, I felt like my life was sort of wrapping up. It seemed like the best part of my life was behind me, and I had only middle and old age ahead. I decided I didn't want to think that way, though, and after getting involved with a menopause support and information site on the Internet, I actually joined a local women's group.

Through the group, I began talking about myself and thinking a lot about my future. The more I talked and listened to others, the more I learned about myself. And the more I learned, the more I began to think about my past and how I got to this place in my life. Looking back at my past helped me to realize the kind of person I am, and the kind of person I'm always going to be. Being part of the group definitely helped me to find a new voice and a new way of seeing myself, but seeing and exploring my past helped me to realize how strong I am and how strong I can be.

IF YOU'VE BEEN working sequentially through this book by now you've covered a lot of ground. You've explored issues about your health and your emotions, and you've thought about what this change means to you, how well you're adjusting to it, and your perspective about the change and yourself.

Now is a good time to take a longer, harder look at yourself. Until this point, you've been focusing on where you are now and where this change might take you. But one way to better understand where you want to go is to look back at where you've been.

Not everybody looks back at their life in pleasure. Not everything has gone just the way it "should" have, and not everyone has accomplished all the things they hoped they would. As people age, they begin to compare themselves with others their own age, and some begin to feel as though time is slipping away. But as you know, menopause is as much about midlife change, self-image, personal growth, and perspective as it is about physical change. When put into this context, it becomes apparent that many of these feelings of uncertainty, self-doubt, and perhaps even inadequacy represent the "meat and potatoes" of middle life development.

Your sense of identity is built on the things you do, your impact on the world, and your perception of your value to others.

Regardless of how "well" you've accomplished earlier tasks, succeeded in earlier relationships, or met career or other personal goals, you have a whole life ahead of you. Your past is the prologue to your future. You have an opportunity to look back and learn from your own history, good and bad, about just who it is you are and who you want to become.

Who Are You?

Questions of personal identity are intimately tied to your future. When asked the generic question, "Who are you?" you're really being asked about who you think you are. This is a question about personal identity—the way you view your role in the world and your relationships with others. Your sense of identity is built on the things you do, your impact on the world, and your perception of your value to others. People with poorly defined identities often are confused about their personal relationships, and the value to others of the things they do, and what's important to them.

In looking back at your past through a journal, you develop a biography or a memoir of your life. The goal in such a task is not to elevate yourself. Instead, it's to help you put your life in perspective and recognize how your past provides the basis on which to build your future. From this point of view, every journal entry in this chapter—every memoir—is intended to help you draw strength and celebrate the person you are today.

Accordingly, the next journal entry is intended only to focus on those positive aspects of who you are *today*. People who struggle to find positive things to look back on or who experience difficulty viewing themselves in a positive light should remember that the basic premise behind this entry is that *everyone* is of value and *everyone* is capable.

The events of your life have given you insight, strength, wisdom, and experience and have thus provided the foundation for the person you are today.

This doesn't mean you have to describe only the most positive or best things that have ever happened to you, but it does mean you have to reach inward to discover how the events of your life have given you insight, strength, wisdom, and experience and have thus provided the foundation for the person you are today. In fact, you may choose to look back at the most difficult moments in your life as those that most helped you to become the person you are today. If you have difficulty with this or any journal entry in this chapter, move ahead to Chapter 9, and then return to work on the entries in this chapter.

Unlike most of the previous journal entries, this next entry calls for free-form style. Other than the questions themselves, little direction is provided. Once again, there is no correct way to complete this entry. Just answer each question in any way that seems most fit, and then take the time to review your answers and think about what you wrote.

THE WELL SPRING

1. Who are you?

_____

_____

_____

_____

_____

_____

2. Where did you come from?

_____

_____

_____

_____

_____

_____

3. What are your greatest strengths?

_____

_____

_____

_____

_____

_____

4. What is the source of your greatest strengths?

_____

_____

_____

_____

_____

_____

_____

_____

5. What were the greatest gifts of your early life?

_____

_____

_____

_____

_____

_____

_____

6. What do you most have to celebrate?

_____

_____

_____

_____

_____

_____

_____

7. How has your past contributed to your present?

_____

_____

_____

_____

_____

_____

_____

_____

8. Complete these sentences.

a. *I was* . . . _____

_____

b. *I am* . . . _____

_____

THINGS TO THINK ABOUT

- Was it difficult working free form or was it liberating, allowing you to write anything you wanted?
- What did you discover about yourself? Do you understand how your past has helped make you the person you are today?
- Is this a journal entry to return to time and time again?

Turning Points

Looking back, there are always moments that stand out as points frozen in time, moments remembered around which change or personal growth seemed to revolve. Sometimes these are moments remembered with great pleasure or joy—the winning of an award, the beginning of a valued relationship, a special trip, or a wonderful day, for example. Sometimes the moment stands out as a clear turning point or change in direction, such as a decision to marry, a career choice, or a path not taken. But not all moments are recalled with pleasure. They may, instead, be tinged with sorrow, anger, or fear. Bad memories, as well as good ones, can become frozen in time. These are the memories of events around which our lives have turned and on which part of the foundation for our current lives is built.

Use the next journal entry to think about important moments and events in your life. Consider moments that stand out in your mind as helping to shape who you became and who you are.

LIFE MARKERS: DEFINING MOMENTS

1. Describe one defining moment in your childhood.

_____

_____

_____

_____

_____

_____

_____

a. Why was this such an important moment?

_____

_____

_____

_____

_____

_____

b. How did this moment contribute to who you are now?

_____

_____

_____

_____

_____

2. Describe one defining moment in your early adolescence.

_____

_____

_____

_____

_____

a. Why was this such an important moment?

_____

_____

_____

_____

_____

b. How did this moment contribute to who you are now?

_____

_____

_____

_____

_____

3. Describe one defining moment in your late adolescence.

_____

_____

_____

_____

_____

_____

_____

a. Why was this such an important moment?

_____

_____

_____

_____

_____

b. How did this moment contribute to who you are now?

_____

_____

_____

_____

_____

4. Describe one defining moment in your early adulthood.

_____

_____

_____

_____

_____

a. Why was this such an important moment?

_____

_____

_____

_____

_____

b. How did this moment contribute to who you are now?

_____

_____

_____

_____

_____

5. Describe one very important moment in your recent life as an adult.

_____

_____

_____

_____

_____

6. How have these events and moments together contributed to help build the person you are today?

_____

_____

_____

_____

_____

Landmark Relationships

Just as there are defining moments in your life, so too are there individuals who, intentionally or otherwise, helped to define your thinking, your personality, and your life. These are the connections, affiliations, and associations that are important not just because they were fun or provided pleasure, but because they contributed in some meaningful way to who you became. These relationships become landmarks that, when you look back at them, served to define your life in some significant way.

Significance is not always the result of a major event. A relationship is not necessarily significant because it was "big." In many instances, people who shaped your life will have had significant relationships with you, but in some cases the life marker may have been a relationship that didn't happen or a passing relationship that quickly moved in and out of your life. Perhaps you count a parent as a person who forever shaped your life, or maybe it was a teacher, or even a fleeting interaction with someone who left a mark on your feelings, your thoughts, and your life long after the interaction ended.

The next journal entry will help you to think about important people and relationships.

Just as there are defining moments in your life, so too are there individuals who, intentionally or otherwise, helped to define your thinking, your personality, and your life.

LIFE MARKERS: PEOPLE

1. List the names and relationships of five important people in your life:

a. _____

b. _____

c. _____

d. _____

e. _____

2. Pick the first person on your list. _____

a. How old were you when this relationship became important, and what were you doing at that time in your life?

_____

_____

b. Why was this person important in your development?

_____

_____

_____

_____

c. How did this relationship influence the person you are today?

_____

_____

_____

_____

3. Pick the second person on your list. _____

a. How old were you when this relationship became important, and what were you doing at that time in your life?

_____

_____

b. Why was this person important in your development?

_____

_____

_____

_____

c. How did this relationship influence the person you are today?

_____

_____

_____

_____

_____

4. Pick the third person on your list. _____

a. How old were you when this relationship became important, and what were you doing at that time in your life?

_____

_____

b. Why was this person important in your development?

_____

_____

_____

_____

c. How did this relationship influence the person you are today?

_____

_____

_____

_____

_____

5. Pick the fourth person on your list. _____

a. How old were you when this relationship became important, and what were you doing at that time in your life?

_____

_____

b. Why was this person important in your development?

_____

_____

_____

c. How did this relationship influence the person you are today?

_____

_____

_____

_____

6. Pick the fifth person on your list. _____

a. How old were you when this relationship became important, and what were you doing at that time in your life?

_____

_____

b. Why was this person important in your development?

_____

_____

_____

c. How did this relationship influence the person you are today?

_____

_____

_____

7. How have these people and relationships together contributed to help build the person you are today?

_____

_____

_____

_____

_____

_____

_____

THINGS TO THINK ABOUT

- Do important people come to mind easily, or is it difficult to get in touch with who most influenced your development?
- Are your memories of important people sweet, bittersweet, or difficult? Is there a pattern of some kind evident in the relationships that most affected and influenced your development?
- Are there important people in your life *today*? Are any of the important people you described still in your life?

A Biography of Your Life

Whereas a biography is written by one person about another, an autobiography is a personal memoir. As you work through this book, you're creating an autobiography of sorts. Your journal contains your ideas and thoughts, your feelings and concerns, and memories of both your past and visions of your future. But a *formal* autobiography or memoir usually has a particular slant or direction and a focus on a specific aspect of the life being chronicled.

Use this next journal entry to create a focused autobiographical sketch of your life. Take only ten minutes. As people are complex beings with rich lives and histories, it's inconceivable that a brief autobiography can do much more than create a character sketch of one aspect of your life. However, because the way you see yourself no doubt varies from day to day and may be influenced by your mood or recent events in your life (or for any number of other reasons), a ten-minute autobiography is likely to capture something important about how you see yourself at the time you wrote it. In other words, a short autobiographical sketch is just as likely to teach you something about yourself right now, as it is to capture some aspect of your past.

A short autobiographical sketch is just as likely to teach you something about yourself right now as it is to capture some aspect of your past.

Describe your life in any way you want. You can focus on your whole life, a single interval in it, or even a single incident. You can write a brief chronological account of your life, or you can shape your autobiography around a theme (for instance, strong influences on your life, memories you've never forgotten, or members of your family). Note that this is a free-form journal entry with little structure to guide you, other than the task itself.

Allow yourself five minutes to think about what you want to write about and how you're going to write it. Then begin writing.

A TEN-MINUTE AUTOBIOGRAPHY

Day: _____   Date: _____

After five minutes' thought and planning, write your autobiography. Time yourself, and write for ten minutes only.

_____

_____

_____

_____

_____

_____

A Second Look

In the previous entry you wrote a ten-minute autobiography. Now look at yourself and your history through a different lens. Pick a different day, and write another ten-minute autobiography without reusing your earlier material. Again, describe your life in any way you want. You can describe your whole life, an interval in your life, or a single incident. You can shape your autobiography on a theme or you can try a free-flowing autobiography.

Should you decide to return to and repeat this journal entry, you can eventually build a complete autobiography of your life through a collection of short essay-style autobiographies that not only record your life as it was, but your life as it is at the time of writing.

ANOTHER TEN-MINUTE AUTOBIOGRAPHY

Day: _____ Date: _____

1. After five minutes' thought and planning, write your additional autobiography. Time yourself, and write for ten minutes only.

_____

_____

2. How is this second autobiography different from your first one?

_____

_____

_____

_____

_____

_____

_____

_____

3. Why is this autobiography different?

_____

_____

_____

_____

_____

_____

4. Would people reading the two autobiographies realize they were reading about the same person?

_____

_____

_____

_____

_____

5. What influenced your choice of material or style for this autobiography?

_____

_____

_____

_____

_____

THINGS TO THINK ABOUT

- How are your two biographies related? Taking both as a whole, what do they say about you as a person?
- Was it difficult or simple to write this second autobiography? Did you discover anything different about yourself?
- Have you learned anything about yourself by writing these biographies? Could you write a third autobiography? Will you?

The Living Autobiography

Writing is a form of self-expression that can help you clarify your thinking and express your feelings, muse out loud to yourself, and capture your life and times on paper.

The next journal entry provides a format for a daily journal entry. This is a simple entry that you can use to unload your thoughts and feelings, describe your day, and record what you're going through as part of your personal history. At the end of the entry, add a thought for the day. This can be anything that impresses, inspires, or strikes you or that in some way is worth remembering. Finding a thought for each day pushes you to look outside yourself, even as you find ways to express what's inside.

A DAILY DIARY

"When I write down my thoughts, they do not escape me. This action makes me remember my strength." — ISIDORE DUCASSE

Day: _____   Date: _____

1. What were the most pressing issues on your mind today?

_____

_____

_____

_____

_____

2. What special tasks, events, or incidents stand out?

_____

_____

_____

_____

_____

3. What did you accomplish today?

_____

_____

_____

_____

_____

_____

4. In general, how were you affected by this day?

_____

_____

_____

_____

_____

_____

5. What is changing over time? Are issues getting resolved or building up?

_____

_____

_____

_____

_____

_____

6. What is going right in your life?

_____

_____

_____

_____

_____

7. Complete these sentences.

a. *Today I'm feeling* . . . _____

_____

_____

b. *I want/need to say* . . . _____

_____

_____

8. Note some other reflections on the day or this time in your life.

_____

_____

_____

_____

_____

THOUGHT FOR THE DAY

_____

_____

_____

_____

_____

THINGS TO THINK ABOUT

• Are there especially difficult days ahead? If so, how can you best prepare for them, and what support do you need?

• Are the days going well? What can you do to improve the chances that they'll keep improving?

• Are there things pressing for you that need your attention? What will happen if they don't get your attention?

The Power of Self-Affirmation

An affirmation is an assertion of a truth, a belief, or an ideal— a way to put out an idea and commit yourself to it.

An affirmation is an assertion of a truth, a belief, or an ideal—a way to put out an idea and commit yourself to it. In this case, the affirmation reflects your commitment to yourself—your own health, goodness, strength, and ability to get through and make the best use of this time in your life. The final journal entry in this chapter provides a means for self-affirmation.

CELEBRATING YOURSELF

1. List at least four things in your life of which you're proud. These can include things you've done or accomplished, children you've parented, relationships you've had, musical instruments you've learned to play, special skills or abilities you've developed, challenges or adversity you've overcome, or decisions you've made.

a. _____

b. _____

c. _____

d. _____

2. Now describe four personal qualities about which you can feel good. These can include your generosity, your intellect, your sense of humor, your organizational skills, your creativity, your compassion for issues or empathy for others, your ability to make new friends, or your attitudes and beliefs.

a. _____

b. _____

c. _____

d. _____

3. Complete these sentences.

a. *I know I can deal with stress and difficulty because I . . .* _____

_____

b. *Even though there are always things to feel badly about, I . . .* _____

_____

c. *Although I'm experiencing changes that are new to me, I . . .* _____

_____

d. *I draw strength from . . .* _____

_____

e. *Above all I value myself because . . .* _____

_____

f. One thought that helps me through difficult times is . . . _____

_____

_____

THINGS TO THINK ABOUT

- Was this a difficult entry for you? Were you able to describe accomplishments or personal qualities of which you're proud? If not, why not?
- Do self-reinforcing thoughts help you gather internal strength or feel better about yourself during a difficult time?
- Will it be useful to focus on a self-affirming thought every day?

9

Destination:
SELF-IMAGE AND
PERSONAL IDENTITY

VICTORIA

I keep myself in great shape, and I still get whistles from the back. But when they see my sixty-year-old face they turn their eyes away. I guess I'll have to start walking backwards anytime I really want to make an impression! Come to think of it, I don't really need it anymore.

LORI

I feel invisible. I used to be conscious of being looked at. Now I'm conscious of not being looked at. Sometimes I like it, sometimes I don't.

NAN

I knew all about empty-nest syndrome, and the idea that your life as a mother and a woman changes when your family grows up. I didn't realize that those parenting changes would combine with changes in my body, my attitudes, and my relationships to really leave me wondering what my role was in the world now that my kids and my husband didn't really need a "mom" anymore. It took me a long time to piece by piece figure out who I was and could be, all over again. It's been great!

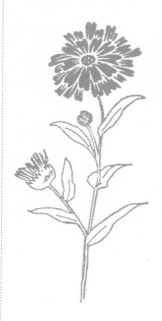

IN A SOCIETY flooded with images of how we should dress, what we should eat and drink, how we should think, and who we should be, it can be difficult to develop a clear sense of who we *would* be if left entirely to our own devices. For women, the issues of personal identity and self-image are especially complex given the inundation of images that inform us of the way women *should* look. These portrayals of women, from Barbie to the anorexic waif, the *Baywatch* babe, the supermodel, and beyond inform women about what is supposedly attractive. From cigarettes to clothing, jewelry, and cosmetics, the media provides an onslaught of images intended to sell women on who they should be or who they should *want* to be.

Self-image is a reflection of how you see yourself.

In this chapter, you'll have a chance to think about who you are by looking at yourself through your own eyes and who you think you might be, seen through the eyes of others. The work in this chapter will help you focus on *changing* self-image and identity.

Self-Image, Personal Identity, and Self-Esteem

Self-image is a reflection of how you see yourself. People with a positive self-image think of themselves as reasonably effective and capable and as someone others would want to know. Personal identity reflects your sense of who you are, or the way you view your role in the world and your relationships with others. Your sense of identity is built on the things you do, your impact on the world, and your perception of your value to others.

People with a negative self-image often see themselves as incapable and perhaps undesirable. People with poorly defined identities often are confused about what's important to them. Self-image has to do with the value you place on yourself; personal identity has more to do with the roles you see yourself playing. One is about your value to your self; the other, your value to those around you. Together they contribute to your sense of self-esteem.

Changing Self-Perception

In the final analysis, self-image, personal identity, and self-esteem are all aspects of self-perception. Hopefully, your self-perception (your sense of who you are) is not influenced too much by the media. Most likely, if you had a high degree of self-esteem, a strong self-image, and a well-defined sense of personal identity before your menopause, things haven't changed too much. It's worth noting that although experiences can weaken your sense of yourself, they can also strengthen self-image, boost self-esteem, and help further develop and solidify personal identity.

Have things changed for you since perimenopause? If so, in which direction, or have you been left unchanged by this event? The next journal entry focuses on the way you see yourself. Because the entry deals with self-concepts, this exercise is a little like looking in a mirror and honestly telling yourself what you think of yourself. Try to answer each question as thoughtfully and as honestly as possible. Remember that this is your journal and your private conversation with yourself. If you find some of your answers difficult to deal with, it may simply signal the beginning of a new openness with yourself.

Self-image has to do with the value you place on yourself; personal identity has more to do with the roles you see yourself playing.

SELF-PERCEPTION

1. Self-Esteem

a. Circle the number that most approximates your sense of self-regard: 1 = feeling pretty lousy about yourself; 5 = feeling pretty great.

Low Self-Esteem			**High Self-Esteem**	
I really feel badly about myself.			I really feel good about myself.	
1	2	3	4	5

b. Explain your rating. How do you feel about yourself, and why?

_____

_____

_____

c. Has your sense of self-esteem changed since perimenopause? If so, how?

_____

_____

_____

2. Self-Image

a. How positive is your self-image?

Negative Self-Image			**Positive Self-Image**	
I see myself as really ineffective.			I see myself as really effective.	
1	2	3	4	5

b. Explain your answer. How do you see yourself, and why?

_____

_____

_____

c. Has your self-image changed since perimenopause? If so, how?

_____

_____

_____

3. Personal Identity

a. How clear is your sense of personal identity?

Confused and Uncertain Identity　　　　**Clear and Certain Identity**

I'm confused or uncertain about my roles.　　I'm clear and certain about my roles.

          1   2   3   4   5

b. Explain your answer. In what ways do you experience confusion or clarity about who you are as a person, both in terms of identity and role?

_____

_____

_____

c. Has your sense of personal identity changed since perimenopause? If so, how?

_____

_____

_____

4. What *is* your overall self-concept? How do you generally see yourself?

_____

_____

_____

_____

5. How much has menopause affected your overall self-concept?

_____

_____

_____

6. What's been the most difficult part of maintaining a healthy self-perception since menopause, and why?

_____

_____

_____

Body Image

Many things affect and influence both self-image and personal identity. Some of these influences were described in Chapter 8. In our society, it isn't possible to talk seriously about women's self-image and identity without discussing body image.

The "ideal" body has varied enormously over time and from culture to culture, but today's ideal female body has been made all too apparent by the media. And with the weight of the average American woman getting heavier and the average Miss America getting taller and thinner each year, the anguish many women feel about their bodies has become palpable.

There are many responses to the physical changes introduced by menopause and this time in your life. For some women, there is a realization that they have consciously or unconsciously counted on being admired physically. For others, there may come relief that it's finally okay to walk down the street and not have to turn heads anymore. This process of change may be more challenging for those whose "beautiful" face and culturally approved body were a critical component of their self-image, even an essential career requirement.

Cultural Image

How people see themselves is often affected by the images presented to them by their culture. Ours is a culture of good looks and, perhaps more to the point, the "right" look. Building a healthy self-image is always a challenge under the best of conditions but, in an environment where looks are valued and self-image is built in part on how attractive you are to others, it is particularly complex. Even if endowed with the kind of face and body that fits the cultural image, you may have to spend a lifetime ensuring that you remain attractive to others, an often increasingly difficult task as you age.

Developing a positive and confident sense of personal identity is also a challenge, especially in a society where your sense of who you are is often intimately tied to your ability to feel or be seen as personally attractive. Although our society is changing, women remain inundated with visions of what it means to be attractive.

How people see themselves is often affected by the images presented to them by their culture.

YOUR BODY, YOURSELF

1. What did you think of your body when . . .

a. you were age thirty?

_____

_____

_____

_____

b. you were age twenty?

_____

_____

_____

_____

c. if you are a mother, when you were pregnant?

_____

_____

_____

_____

2. What do you think about the body you have *now*?

_____

_____

_____

_____

a. What are the features you like the most?

_____

_____

_____

_____

b. What are the features you like the least?

_____

_____

_____

_____

3. What are the differences between your *own* body image and the cultural image of how your body *should* look?

_____

_____

_____

_____

4. If there are differences between your body image and the cultural image, how can you best deal with those differences?

_____

_____

_____

_____

_____

5. Will the ways you choose to deal with the differences enhance or damage your self-image?

_____

_____

_____

_____

_____

6. How much does cultural image affect your self-image?

_____

_____

_____

_____

_____

7. How much does cultural image affect your sense of personal identity?

_____

_____

_____

_____

_____

8. What do you think of the cultural image?

_____

_____

_____

_____

_____

_____

THINGS TO THINK ABOUT

- Should cultural images of women dictate or affect the way you see your own body?
- Should you make changes in your appearance and body image because of the cultural image? Would you consider making changes if not for cultural image?
- If you are going to make changes, what changes can you reasonably make? How will you begin the process of change?

Self-Image and Personal Identity in the Real World

It would be great if it were enough to just think good and positive thoughts about yourself in order to have a positive self-image and strong sense of personal identity. But it just isn't that simple. Because we're social beings, what we think of ourselves (self-image) and our sense of who we are (personal identity) is intimately tied to our personal relationships and general interactions with others. Although most people would, perhaps, like to see their self-image as strong and unaffected by others, it's nonetheless true that our interactions and communication with others do affect and help shape our sense of who we are. In other words, we're dependent on one another not only for the basic necessities of life but also for our sense of personal identity, success, and importance. It's not that social interactions and transactions alone define who we are, but they're certainly important.

We're dependent on one another not only for the basic necessities of life, but also for our sense of personal identity, success, and importance.

CONNECTIONS

1. How much does your self-esteem, self-image, and personal identity depend on the way you're seen by others?

_____

_____

_____

_____

_____

2. What sort of interactions with others do you most need to help boost your self-esteem?

_____

_____

_____

_____

_____

3. What sort of things do you most need from others to confirm or define a healthy self-image?

_____

_____

_____

_____

_____

4. What sort of support do you most need from others to help shape and develop a clear personal identity?

_____

_____

_____

_____

5. In general, what do you need from your personal relationships?

_____

_____

_____

_____

_____

6. Are your personal relationships . . .

a. satisfying? Do they help build a sense of self-worth and personal meaning in your life?

_____

_____

_____

b. supportive? Do they help you understand, deal with, and get through this time of change?

_____

_____

_____

c. understanding? Do they offer you the level of intimacy, familiarity, and sensitivity that you most need as you deal with the issues of menopause?

_____

_____

_____

7. Do you share enough of your experiences and your needs with the people closest to you?

_____

_____

_____

_____

_____

THINGS TO THINK ABOUT

- Should you share more with the people closest to you? Do you need to share more? What most prevents you from telling people what you want or need?
- Are you clear on how relationships and personal interactions affect your sense of self?
- Are you clear on the differences between self-esteem, self-image, and personal identity?

Focusing on Self

As you deal with issues of self-esteem and personal identity, you're dealing with some of the most complex issues facing women in our society today. Who are you, what's your role, who do you want to be, and who can you be? Despite the reality that many of these large issues are affected by and evolve in the context of our larger society, the immediate and most personal aspects of these questions come down to you. Think of these same questions, then, not from a social and more global point of view but from a strictly limited and entirely personal perspective: who are *you*, what's *your* role, who do *you* want to be, and who *can you* be?

By now, you realize that menopause provides the opportunity to cultivate a new kind of self-image, self-respect, and personal identity. In this chapter, you've dealt with not only concepts of self as they exist in your mind but also the effect of culture and social relationships on self-image. But as all your experiences are filtered through your mind, it is your perceptions, feelings, thoughts, and ideas that count. All those things going on in your life right now, and the way you're making sense of and dealing with those things, have a powerful influence on your body. Accordingly, thinking about and recognizing what you most value right now, about yourself and your life, is a powerful tool to promote a healthy body, a healthy mind, and a healthy self-image for your future.

If you've been working sequentially through this book, you're by now squarely in the third stage of your journey—focusing on self—and moving toward the final stage. Use the final entry in this chapter to consider these questions of self-image and identity, and the related issues.

CHECKPOINT: FOCUSING ON YOURSELF

1. How much does your self-esteem, self-image, and personal identity depend on others in your life?

_____

_____

_____

_____

_____

2. How do you deal with the pressures to conform to an image created for you by someone else?

_____

_____

_____

_____

3. What are three barriers in your life right now to a healthy self-image and a well-defined sense of personal identity?

a. _____

b. _____

c. _____

4. What are three things you can positively do to . . .

a. boost self-esteem? _____

_____

_____

b. maintain healthy self-image? _____

_____

_____

c. build personal identity?_____

_____

_____

5. Write five positive self-affirming statements about yourself at this time in your life:

a. *I am* . . . _____

_____

_____

b. *I am* . . . _____

_____

_____

c. *I am* . . . _____

_____

_____

d. *I am* . . . _____

_____

_____

e. *I am* . . . _____

_____

_____

THINGS TO THINK ABOUT

- Were you easily able to come up with five self-affirming statements? If so, what does this tell you about yourself? If not, what does this tell you? Do you need some help figuring out how to best boost self-esteem?
- Do you have the kind of supports, structures, and relationships in your life to productively and successfully work through menopausal and other midlife experiences? Do you need to work on developing a stronger personal support system?
- Are you a "victim" of cultural expectations, or are you the shaper of your own destiny?

10

Destination:

CONTEMPLATION AND

REFLECTION

"With an eye made quiet by the power Of harmony, and the deep power of joy, We see into the life of things."
—WILLIAM WORDSWORTH

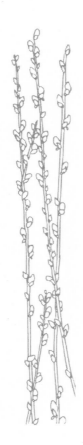

MARIE

It was difficult to see beyond big changes at first. My menopause came early, brought on by a hysterectomy. That took me off my feet for weeks, and I felt depressed for quite some time afterwards. Although I had one child, I wanted more and I felt like my life had been taken out of my hands. After a while I decided to see a counselor, and that really helped me think differently about things. I learned to take another approach to my life, and look at things from another perspective. I came to realize that although we couldn't have another child, we could adopt. That was not only two (adopted) children ago, but it was also the start of a new way of thinking for me.

GRACE

I read a lot about menopause once I realized it was happening to me. I can't really say enough about how much I got from what I read. It was as though a whole new door opened, allowing me to see myself and my life in an entirely different way. My life today, after menopause, is a lot more focused and more genuine in many ways than it was before. Is that the result of hormonal change, the wis-

dom of middle age, or just a change in attitude? I don't know, but I sure feel like I understand myself more.

ANITA BROOKNER, THE British novelist, said, "What is interesting about self-analysis is that it leads nowhere—it is an art form in itself." This, perhaps, is the essence of contemplation and reflection: the art of simply looking inside, and through that inner search understanding more about yourself *and* the world. The words of Franz Kafka build on this idea: "It is not necessary that you leave the house. Remain at your table and listen. Do not even listen, only wait. Do not even wait, be wholly still and alone. The world will present itself to you for its unmasking."

In this chapter, you'll have the opportunity to stop and listen to yourself, to see the world around you in a different way, and perhaps learn to see yourself in a different way too.

Reflection

Contemplation means exploring feelings without passion, considering the world without taking action, and speaking to yourself without words.

Reflection is a perfect word to describe the essential quality of this third stage of the menopausal journey, as the focus of your attention moves tightly around yourself. It's important to be able to take a deep breath, slow things down, and examine each piece of life through the new eyes that reflection and contemplation can provide. Slowing down means stepping outside your daily life for a moment or two and, from this quieter and slower place, considering the world in which you live and *how* you live in it, discovering for yourself what has value and what works best for you. The goal is to simply think about things for which you don't always have answers. Contemplation means exploring feelings without passion, considering the world without taking action, and speaking to yourself without words. This act of looking inside helps you know yourself and understand how you affect and are affected by the world outside.

People contemplate in many different ways: a solitary walk or a bicycle ride in the mountains; a hot bath with soothing music playing quietly in the background; a daily journal entry exploring the complexities, thoughts, and events of the day; dancing or painting or allowing yourself to be carried away by a piece of poetry. For some, contemplation means closing their eyes to the outside world and reflecting on a thought or idea.

But not everyone is naturally contemplative. For some, slowing down and thinking in this way is just not part of their normal way of doing things. Nevertheless, at this critical time in your life and personal development, contemplation is an important tool to develop, learn, and use.

Getting Inspired

The history of literature and recorded thought is also the history of ideas: the words of wisdom and the encapsulation of the human experience. For this reason, many turn to quotations and verse to summarize and reflect the ideas and experiences of those who have stepped this way before. At the beginning of each chapter of this book and in many other places within the text, you've found quotations that are intended sometimes to inspire, sometimes to educate, sometimes to capsulize an idea or experience, and sometimes to help put things into perspective.

The words of others, whether quotations, verses of poetry, excerpts from essays or books, or snippets of speeches have tremendous power.

The words of others, whether quotations, verses of poetry, excerpts from essays or books, or snippets of speeches have tremendous power. They put us in touch with the entire human experience or a moment of experience especially relevant to our lives. For the next journal entry, first look back through this book at those quotations that hold special meaning for you, or turn to any other source of words that inspire you. People are moved by songs, poetry, speeches, letters, and entire volumes containing only quotations are available for your perusal.

WORDS OF WISDOM

1. Select three favorite or otherwise meaningful quotations, and copy each here.

a. _____

_____

b. _____

_____

c. _____

_____

2. Pick one of these quotations for this entry, and describe what made you select this particular quotation for this entry.

_____

_____

_____

_____

3. How do these words have relevance to your life at this time?

_____

_____

_____

_____

_____

4. What do these words mean to you?

_____

_____

_____

_____

_____

5. In what ways can these words instruct you or offer you direction?

_____

_____

_____

_____

_____

THINGS TO THINK ABOUT

- Were you able to find three quotations that moved you? Was it easy or difficult to find sources for them?
- Were you able to understand why the quotation you chose moved you?
- Did you find meaning in the entry? Will you repeat it for the other two quotations you chose? Will you continue to search out the words of others?

Looking Around

Look around you. Look at the things that surround you: magazines, television, movies, newspapers, popular fiction and nonfiction, the evening news, talk shows, advertisements, the Internet. Take a closer look.

Media comprise all those things that communicate ideas to us and through which ideas are passed. Many people feel that the media don't just pass on ideas to us but actually add and communicate messages of their own. Look carefully at the media that surround you. Before starting the next journal entry, spend the next three days paying special attention to the media through which ideas are passed on to you.

In this journal entry, after you've answered the first five questions, create a collage based on how you experience the media in your life. A collage is a collection of bits and pieces of flat objects such as magazine photographs, newspapers, pressed flowers, fabric, ticket stubs, and so on that are pasted together to form a piece of artwork. Sometimes the various pieces are juxtaposed to show contrast or differing ideas, sometimes to reflect or express a particular idea or emotion. Include in your collage anything you want, from your present or your past, but as the organizing theme use your experiences with the media in your life and what you've learned from your closer observations.

LISTENING TO THE MEDIA

1. What media did you concentrate on? Check all that apply.

__advertisements   __magazines   __newspapers

__books, fiction   __movies   __radio

__books, nonfiction   __music   __talk shows

__Internet   __news shows   __television

other: _____   _____

_____   _____

_____   _____

_____   _____

_____   _____

_____   _____

2. What did the media tell you about social attitudes regarding . . .

a. alcohol?_____

_____

_____

b. business and finance?_____

_____

_____

c. celebrityhood? _____

_____

_____

d. eating and food? _____

_____

_____

e. fashion and style? _____

_____

_____

f. lifestyle? _____

_____

_____

g. morality? _____

_____

_____

h. privacy? _____

_____

_____

i. privilege? _____

_____

_____

j. relationships? _____

_____

_____

k. sexuality and sexual relationships? _____

_____

_____

l. social values? _____

_____

_____

m. women? _____

_____

_____

n. men? _____

_____

_____

3. What did you learn from your closer observation of the media?

_____

_____

_____

_____

4. Do the media represent your lifestyle, values, or opinions?

_____

_____

_____

_____

5. What can you learn about your society and culture through the media?

_____

_____

_____

_____

_____

CREATE YOUR COLLAGE IN THIS SPACE OR ON A SEPARATE SHEET OF PAPER

7. Look at your collage.

a. What does your collage tell you about your response and attitude toward the media?

_____

_____

_____

_____

_____

_____

b. What does your collage say about your view of your world?

_____

_____

_____

_____

_____

c. What does your collage tell you about *you*?

_____

_____

_____

_____

_____

_____

8. Give your collage a title.

_____

Rediscovering Your Life

People tread the same paths every day: the same relationships, the same interactions, the same tasks, and the same routines. When we see the same things every day, two things may become invisible to us. First, we may stop seeing those things that are so usual and commonplace that they're just "always" there. These are the things we take for granted—they're routine. It's not that they're not important; it's just that we become blind to them and sometimes their value. Second, we may miss seeing things that are just off the regular track. We fail to see them not because we take them for granted, but because we're simply not looking.

When we see the same things every day, two things may become invisible to us.

In many ways, the essence of contemplation is the deliberate study of the usual in order to find something new. Within your own life, there are probably many things and many relationships you've stopped seeing or that are tucked so far away that you've almost forgotten about them. There are probably also many unexplored corners, many things you've never noticed or thought about, and many unexamined clues to how you've lived your life and how you *want* to live it now. One way to become more aware of your life, and what's going on around you and inside of you, is to find time each day to stop and think. The next journal entry provides a means for a daily search of your life and the opportunity to reflect each day on what you've learned about yourself from that search.

In this journal entry you'll build a portrait of yourself over seven days, based on the things in your daily life. Each day, you'll embark on a search within your everyday life for those things that are always there. In some cases, it will be simple to locate search items; other times, you may have to stretch your mind. Items that were easy to find on Day 1 may be considerably more difficult to find by Day 7. Remember, you're not looking for earth-shattering realizations, but for the ordinary things and relationships that make up your life.

The exercise runs over a seven-day period, concluding each evening with a written journal entry that summarizes your day. You'll need a small notebook that you can easily keep with you during the day to jot down your thoughts and your discoveries as you search for each item. You'll also need a small camera that you can carry with you each day. A cheap, disposable camera will suffice.

For each day of the seven days, find:

- *Something important in your life.* Find something in your *daily* life that has special meaning to you. A possession or article of clothing, a piece of jewelry or memento of some kind, a photograph or painting, or an important event or ritual that's part of your everyday life. Here you may find yourself looking at the very things you normally take for granted.

- *An interesting corner of your life.* Find some physical aspect of your life, something that's always there but you never normally see because you're not normally looking for it: a fascinating play of light and shadow through a window at a certain time of day, the way the trees outside of your window move in the breeze, the way two walls in your home or office intersect to create an interesting angle, or the pattern on an armchair or wallpaper.

- *A token or symbol of your life.* Find something in your life that serves as a symbol of who you are, your identity, or your achievements. This could be something you intentionally wear or carry each day to make a statement about yourself or your beliefs or something that unintentionally says something about you or your life.

- *A photograph of your life.* For each day of this journal entry, take one photograph. Your goal is to see things through creative eyes and to look for an opportunity each day to take a snapshot of something in your life that moves you or says something about yourself and your life. It can be a photograph of a corner of your house, a street sign, a person you know, a self-portrait, or clouds in the sky.

- *A choice in your life.* As you move through your days, you make choices, many without thought. During each day of this journal exercise, consider the choices you're making, such as drinking an extra cup of coffee, or staying an extra hour at work, and consider all the things you're choosing to *not* do, such as walk the dog, mow the lawn, or get some exercise.

- *A reflection about your life.* The daily journal entry ends each day with an observation about yourself and what you've learned from the search of your life you've conducted that day.

At the end of each day, briefly describe the items you discovered.

At the end of each day, briefly describe the items you discovered. Include a brief description of the photograph you took for the day. You can later add the photos to your journal, if you choose. At the completion of the seven days write a concluding entry that summarizes your experience with this journal entry.

THE UNDISCOVERED WORLD

DAY 1

Something important in my life: _____

An interesting corner of my life: _____

A token or symbol of my life: _____

A photograph of my life: _____

A choice in my life: _____

Reflection on my search for this day:

_____

_____

_____

_____

_____

_____

DAY 2

Something important in my life: _____

An interesting corner of my life: _____

A token or symbol of my life: _____

A photograph of my life: _____

A choice in my life: _____

Reflection on my search for this day:

_____

_____

_____

_____

_____

DAY 3

Something important in my life: _____

An interesting corner of my life: _____

A token or symbol of my life: _____

A photograph of my life: _____

A choice in my life: _____

Reflection on my search for this day:

_____

_____

_____

_____

_____

_____

_____

DAY 4

Something important in my life: _____

An interesting corner of my life: _____

A token or symbol of my life: _____

A photograph of my life: _____

A choice in my life: _____

Reflection on my search for this day:

_____

_____

_____

_____

_____

_____

_____

DAY 5

Something important in my life: _____

An interesting corner of my life: _____

A token or symbol of my life: _____

A photograph of my life: _____

A choice in my life: _____

Reflection on my search for this day:

_____

_____

_____

_____

_____

_____

DAY 6

Something important in my life: _____

An interesting corner of my life: _____

A token or symbol of my life: _____

A photograph of my life: _____

A choice in my life: _____

Reflection on my search for this day:

_____

_____

_____

_____

_____

_____

DAY 7

Something important in my life: _____

An interesting corner of my life: _____

A token or symbol of my life: _____

A photograph of my life: _____

A choice in my life: _____

Reflection on my search for this day:

_____

_____

_____

_____

_____

_____

_____

Answer these final questions only after you've completed all seven days of the exercise.

1. What have you learned about your life from this seven-day entry?

_____

_____

_____

_____

_____

2. What have you learned about yourself?

_____

_____

_____

_____

_____

3. How can you use this portrait of your life to help open your eyes to fresh ideas?

_____

_____

_____

_____

_____

THINGS TO THINK ABOUT

- Did you discover anything new and interesting about yourself?
- Do you need to be more open to new ways of seeing and thinking? How can you build a fresh perspective into your life?
- Was there anything disturbing about this entry?

You Can See a Lot Just by Looking

A walk puts you back in control—of the pace at which you move, where you go, and what you see.

Walking is a wonderful way to accomplish a great many things. A brisk walk provides exercise, and a slow walk offers an alternative to a usually fast-paced life. It takes you out of the insulated world of your car or the bus and puts you directly into your environment. A solitary walk takes you away from the crowds, interactions, and chatter of everyday life. In many ways, a walk puts you back in control—of the pace at which you move, where you go, and what you see.

The next journal entry will both help to slow you down and open you up to what's around you. It can help you to see those things that you normally may not notice because they're in the background of your life, invisible because you simply aren't looking for them. This entry is intended to direct your attention to the outward and the inward, to use your environment to help you find new and refreshing ways to think.

Take a walk of your choice—along a city street, across a beach, through a park or the woods, or anywhere else you'd like. But go alone, and spend at least thirty minutes on your walk. Walk slowly, and think about yourself and your surroundings, drinking in everything around you: the sounds, the images, and the smells. Take a notebook and a pen with you. If you look, listen, and think, you'll notice all sorts of things that you might not have seen before, and you will have found a way to tune in to those ordinary things around you that can provide pleasure, comfort, and meaning. If you can apply these skills on your walk, you can learn to use them in your everyday life as well. Read the next two journal entries *before* you leave for your walk, and perhaps jot them down in your notebook. Be prepared to write the entire time you're on your walk. Every time you're struck by a smell, sight, sound, or a thought, write it down. After your walk is over, complete the next two journal entries.

THE ROAD NOT TAKEN

Two roads diverged in a wood, and I—
I took the one less traveled by,
And that has made all the difference.
—ROBERT FROST

1. Where did you walk?

_____

_____

_____

_____

_____

2. Why did you choose this particular walk?

_____

_____

_____

3. Describe your walk.

_____

_____

_____

a. *I walked along* . . . _____

b. *I walked through* . . . _____

c. *Along the way, I* . . . _____

4. Describe the weather that day.

_____

_____

_____

5. Think about what you noticed on your walk.
a. What colors stood out the most for you, and why?

_____

_____

_____

b. What sounds could you pick out, near and far?

_____

_____

_____

_____

c. What odors or scents were carried in the air? Were they familiar smells? What did these smells make you think of?

_____

_____

_____

_____

_____

d. What interesting textures did you stop and feel?

_____

_____

_____

_____

_____

6. What did you notice on this walk that you never noticed before?

_____

_____

_____

_____

_____

7. What did you think about on your walk?

_____

_____

_____

_____

_____

Change

Change is inevitable and part of nature. Things constantly change from one state into another. Sometimes the transformation is complete, and all traces of the thing that once existed seem to disappear. At other times, the past is incorporated into and evident in the change. Change is the reason you're keeping this journal.

This next journal entry builds on your walk and has you think about the changes you noticed along the way. The type and rapidity of changes will depend, of course, on *where* you walked. If you walked along the artificially constructed streets of a city or suburban environment, you'll see signs of changes that have occurred pretty routinely and quickly. In contrast, if you walked along a remote mountaintop, you'll have observed the sort of changes that have taken place almost unnoticeably over thousands of years, mostly by erosion and other natural forces. If you walked through woods, you may have noticed a contrast between changes brought by civilization, such as trails and intentionally planted trees, and natural changes as the woods overcome these artificial changes by simply absorbing or growing over them. Use the entry to consider the meaning of change and the delicate balance that exists between change and stasis.

THE DELICATE BALANCE

1. What evidence of change did you see on your walk?

_____

_____

_____

_____

_____

2. Were some changes permanent and others temporary?

_____

_____

_____

_____

3. How did change contribute to the environment?

_____

_____

_____

_____

_____

4. What did change rob from the environment?

_____

_____

_____

_____

5. Was change in the environment of your walk inevitable?

_____

_____

_____

_____

_____

6. Was change necessary?

_____

_____

_____

_____

_____

7. What if no change had occurred in this environment?

_____

_____

_____

_____

_____

_____

8. What if there were *only* change?

_____

_____

_____

_____

_____

_____

Meaning Through Discovery

There's meaning everywhere. Some people look around and find meaning everywhere in their lives; others search and search but fail to find meaning in any corner of their lives. The ability to find meaning is within us and is perhaps part of the human condition. The work that you've completed in this chapter has given you new eyes through which to explore and experience your world and find meaning within it.

Some people look around and find meaning everywhere in their lives.

11

Destination:
TAKING STOCK OF
YOUR LIFE

*"The real meditation is
. . . the meditation on
one's* identity. . . . *You
try finding out why
you're you and not
somebody else. And who
in the blazes are you
anyhow?"*
——EZRA POUND

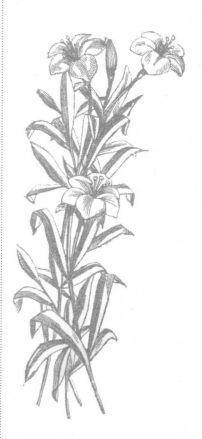

ELISE

*One day, I was struck by the fact that I'd never really considered my
own life as having an end. I knew it intellectually, of course, but
when I turned fifty it was a different kind of acknowledgment. Even
if I planned another healthy forty years, I was on the downward
slope of my life.*

*I'd never understood my mother's laughter at the comedian Jack
Benny's joke about perennially remaining thirty-nine, and I'd never
thought about phrases like "over the hill." But although I was still
actively involved in family and work and didn't feel "middle-aged,"
my perspective on life shifted, and it never returned to what it was
before. It wasn't what's often called "midlife crisis," but it was an
important transformation in my whole sense of what was important
in my life. In a way, I found it very liberating.*

PERHAPS IT'S THE sore back after raking leaves or the injury that
once took several days to heal, but now lingers on for weeks or
even months. Perhaps you first notice the change when you have
to hold a book at arm's length to read the print clearly. It may be

the general aches and pains that once weren't there, the graying hair, or the extra weight that just won't go away. These are the physical changes that affect us all, men and women, at some point between ages thirty-five and sixty. These physical changes in turn signal the emotional issues and questions related to middle age: that we have reached the midpoint of our life, the "end" of our youth, and the swing toward our later years. This transitional period sets the pace for what lies ahead.

Menopause falls in the middle of your life, which is a vastly different situation than that faced by your grandmothers, and perhaps even your mothers, whose life expectancy after menopause was comparatively short. The quality of health and life available has also improved with each generation. Beyond the physical, emotional, and spiritual changes related specifically to menopause itself, there are also broader changes associated with getting older. At this time in your life, you face the real issues of who you are and who you're going to be. Perhaps the most critical issue is not to "recover" from, overcome, or get through menopause and the midlife years but rather to use this significant and important change of life as a jumping-off point for the rest of your life and as an opportunity to further define a strong identity and fortify yourself for the many years of rewarding life ahead. This is not about holding on to youth but instead using your history as the basis for your future.

The need to sit back and take stock is described by Naomi Lucks and Melene Smith in *A Woman's Midlife Companion*. They write, "We can't avoid making the midlife journey, but we can plan our own itinerary. We can use the 'pause' in menopause to stop for a moment and survey the terrain, check out the many paths, and pick up the reins of our own lives. We can honor the many changes of midlife for what they are: the biological event that marks a profound life transition, a wake-up call to the chance to live our lives as fully and deeply as possible."

Beyond the physical, emotional, and spiritual changes related specifically to menopause, there are also broader changes associated with getting older.

Paths to Midlife

There are many paths to midlife. All are different, but each intersects at a point in midlife where women may ask themselves how they got here and where they are going now. Of course, not all women face these anxious midlife experiences. Your path is your own, and whatever your circumstances, the path you took —including the thoughts, feelings, wishes, fantasies, images, and desires that tug at *your* consciousness—is well worth thinking about.

Use this journal entry to describe your path into midlife. The free-writing format of the entry will help you think about and formulate your story.

YOUR PATH TO MIDLIFE

1. Briefly tell your story. Describe your path from early womanhood to menopause and midlife.

_____

_____

_____

_____

_____

_____

_____

_____

_____

_____

_____

_____

_____

2. When were you first aware of being a woman rather than a girl?

_____

_____

_____

_____

3. When were you first aware of your sexuality?

_____

_____

_____

_____

4. Were your early experiences in womanhood satisfying or frustrating?

_____

_____

_____

_____

5. Looking back, did you take charge of your own life and your own womanhood, or were you simply carried along by the events of your life?

_____

_____

_____

_____

_____

6. Did midlife just sneak up on you without warning? Did you ever think it would really arrive?

_____

_____

_____

_____

_____

_____

_____

7. When and how did you first become aware of the arrival of midlife?

_____

_____

_____

_____

_____

8. Are you getting carried kicking and screaming into midlife, accepting midlife graciously, or looking forward to and appreciating the changes that midlife will bring?

_____

_____

_____

_____

_____

_____

_____

Taking Inventory of Your Life

What are the important things in your life, the things that enrich and add to it, make it comfortable, inject meaning, provide the impetus to go on, and, ultimately, make it satisfying and interesting? Many related issues and ideas have been covered in other chapters (you may wish to review, for instance, Chapters 5, 8, 9, and 10), but now is the time to put together some of these ideas, especially in connection with what you *already* know about your life.

The ability and willingness to step outside of daily life and develop a new and different perspective becomes an important component in examining the molds we form for ourselves.

Life is filled with many possibilities, though they often become obscured by midlife when familiar routines become entrenched. Life just *is*, for many people: expectations are set, responsibilities defined, and a pattern ingrained. The ability and willingness to step outside daily life and develop a new and different perspective becomes an important component in examining the molds we form for ourselves. The reminder to examine our lives periodically and take inventory of what we have, what we want, and what we no longer need offers a wonderful opportunity to refresh, refurbish, and renew our lives. In this way we may grow older, but we don't allow ourselves or our thinking to stagnate.

Use the next journal entry to take an inventory of your life. Bear in mind, however, that no journal entry can ever be "complete." A journal is a running documentary of your life, not just one moment in time. The goal of all of the journal entries in this book is to stimulate your thinking and help you move in a direction where you'll keep looking at your life, your needs, and your ideas. Accordingly, this entry is intended to help spark a review and honest appraisal of your life.

TAKING STOCK OF YOUR LIFE

1. What's important in your life? Check every area that's important.
Relationships with:

__children   __coworkers   __friends   __family   __spouse/partner/lover

other: _____   _____

__adventure   __education   __home life   __profession

__career   __fun   __independence   __security

__community   __hobbies/pursuits __physical health __travel

other: _____   _____

_____   _____

_____   _____

2. Look back on the items you've checked off. Is there a pattern? Are most of these items compatible with one another, or do some represent contradictions and conflicts?

_____

_____

_____

_____

_____

_____

_____

3. What are the most important things in your life?

_____

_____

_____

_____

_____

4. What are the most satisfying things in your life?

_____

_____

_____

_____

_____

5. What's missing in your life right now?

_____

_____

_____

_____

_____

6. What do you envision in your future life that's missing now?

_____

_____

_____

_____

_____

7. Are you satisfied with your life?

_____

_____

_____

_____

_____

_____

8. Now look back at the items you checked off in Question 1. Are you paying genuine attention to each of these areas to keep their importance alive and vital, or are you taking each area for granted?

_____

_____

_____

_____

_____

_____

_____

9. What have you learned about your current life from this inventory?

_____

_____

_____

_____

_____

_____

_____

_____

Relationships

Relationships are central in any life. They are the connecting point between ourselves and the rest of the world; they make us *socially* human. Although there's more focus on relationships in Chapter 12, this is a good starting point to begin taking stock of your life and of your relationships, specifically, the quality of them.

TAKING STOCK OF YOUR RELATIONSHIPS

1. Are you satisfied with your relationships?

_____

_____

_____

_____

2. What do you most want from your relationships? Check all that apply.

__adventure	__intellectual stimulation	__sense of being needed
__comfort	__intimacy	__sense of importance
__companionship	__love	__sense of being valued
__family	__recognition	__sex
__friendship	__respect	__understanding
__fun	__safety	__warmth

other: _____   _____

_____   _____

_____   _____

3. Review what you've just checked off. Summarize your relationship needs.

_____

_____

_____

_____

4. List your three greatest needs from your relationships.

a. _____

b. _____

c. _____

5. List your three greatest frustrations with your relationships.

a. _____

b. _____

c. _____

6. What are the most satisfying relationships in your life?

_____

_____

_____

_____

7. What are the least satisfying?

_____

_____

_____

_____

8. Think carefully about each phrase below, and complete the sentences honestly, even though you may not like your answers.

a. *My relationships are . . .* _____

_____

b. *When I think of the sort of relationships I have, I . . .* _____

_____

c. *With my relationships, I most need to work on . . .* _____

_____

d. *If there's one thing I need to change in my relationships, it's . . .* _____

_____

e. *When it comes to my relationships, I need . . .* _____

_____

THINGS TO THINK ABOUT

• Was this a "searching and fearless" inventory of your relationships? If not, what held you back? If it was, how does your relationship inventory leave you feeling?

• Are you satisfied with your relationships? Is this an area to work on changing and improving in your changing life?

• What have you learned about yourself and your life through reviewing your relationships?

Stress and Relaxation

One of the things that most interferes with our ability to see clearly, make good decisions, and plan for the future is stress. It's not that stress is necessarily bad. Stress is a necessary and positive aspect of life since it can create the kind of tension needed to actually hold things together and often pushes us toward change.

Even under the best of circumstances, however, stress is a pressure that must be managed. Although stress may serve to remind or warn us of the need to make change, sound decisions are usually not made under stress. As you consider your past, present, and future, and you move toward and into the fourth and final stage of this journey, it will be important to make decisions from a place free of stress. Your goal is stress management and relaxation. In the beginning of this book, the very first journal entry emphasized finding the time to relax so you could consider the world from a different vantage point. You may want to repeat that entry now. (The purpose, remember, is to use that exercise regularly so that you can learn to find breathing space and build it into your daily life.)

The ability to relax is important to good physical and mental health. The inability to relax can carry a big price tag: physical and emotional fatigue, tension and stress, worry and anxiety, and a constant state of being on the edge. Use the following brief journal entry to think about your ability to relax and manage stress.

Although stress may serve to remind or warn us of the need to make change, sound decisions are usually not made under stress.

TAKING STOCK OF STRESS AND RELAXATION

1. What are the greatest areas of stress in your life right now?

_____

_____

_____

_____

_____

2. Check off methods you use to relax and those techniques that might help if you used them. Add others below. In addition, include your use of alcohol or drugs, prescribed or over-the-counter medications, or other things you do to help relax, even if you're depending on ways to relax that are self-destructive or otherwise potentially harmful. Be honest.

__alcohol	__meditation	__self-hypnosis	__walking
__breathing control	__prescription medicine	__sports	__warm bath
__cigarettes	__quiet music	__talking	__writing
__cup of tea	__reading	__television	__yoga, tai chi,
__drugs	__relaxation tapes	__visualization	etc.

other: _____   _____

_____   _____

_____   _____

3. Look back at the items you just checked off. Are any of your preferred ways to relax problematic?

_____

_____

_____

_____

_____

4. What can you do to learn to relax more completely?

_____

_____

_____

_____

THINGS TO THINK ABOUT

- Is relaxing a problem for you? What most interferes with your ability to relax? How can you overcome these obstacles?
- Do others ever express a concern that you don't relax enough, or you relax in ways that are unhealthy?
- Do you need to change some aspect of your lifestyle in order to take better care of your emotional and physical health?

Realizing Choice

Menopause is not a choice you make. But you do have choices about how to handle menopause. If you get only one thing from this book, hopefully it will be the realization that you always have choices, even in menopause and midlife.

Choice, of course, is relative. Sometimes your choices are wide open, restricted by only your imagination and your will. At other times, your choices are limited by your circumstances. For a single woman with no long-term debts or responsibilities, almost anything goes. On the other hand, if you're forty-five years old with three young children, a heavy mortgage, and few discretionary funds, your choices may be far more limited. Although current circumstances can prevent immediate choice, people are still able to overcome their present situation and work toward change over time. In other words, although your life is no doubt limited by many real-life constraints over which you don't necessarily have full control, it doesn't mean you can't make choices. At this juncture in your life, your choices are not about what you did in the past or even about what you choose to do today. They're about what you can do with your life now and what you're going to do tomorrow.

Your daily life, experience of the world, and even *important aspects* of your identity are largely defined by these four major components:

Although current circumstances can prevent immediate choice, people are still able to overcome their present situation and work toward change over time.

1. *Vocational choices.* These are the activities you do, such as work, school, volunteer work, home making, and so on, that help define your identity.

2. *Social activities.* These are the personal activities in which you engage.

3. *Relationships.* These are the people in whom you invest your personal energy and with whom you spend time, whether platonically or romantically.

4. *Lifestyle.* This includes where and how you live, and the tasks and responsibilities of your everyday life.

Your daily responsibilities may be defined by your role as a parent, for instance, or by your work.

Some of these things may be unchangeable or highly resistant to change. Your daily responsibilities may be defined by your role as a parent, for instance, or by your work. Although you can't stop being a parent, you can nevertheless change at least some of the circumstances that affect your life and ability to make choices. Use the final journal entry in this chapter to think about the possibility of change.

TAKING STOCK OF CHANGE

1. Complete these sentences.

a. *In my life, I'm most satisfied with* . . . _____

_____

b. *In my life, I'm least satisfied with* . . . _____

_____

c. *I would most like to change* . . . _____

_____

d. *I wish I could* . . . _____

_____

2. Consider your current vocation.
a. How satisfied are you?

_____

_____

b. Are there changes you'd like to make?

_____

_____

c. What stops you from making changes?

_____

_____

3. Consider your social activities.
a. How satisfied are you?

_____

_____

b. Are there changes you'd like to make?

_____

_____

c. What stops you from making changes?

_____

_____

4. Consider your relationships.
a. How satisfied are you?

_____

_____

b. Are there changes you'd like to make?

_____

_____

c. What stops you from making changes?

_____

_____

5. Consider your lifestyle.
a. How satisfied are you?

_____

_____

b. Are there changes you'd like to make?

_____

_____

c. What stops you from making changes?

_____

_____

6. What areas of your life are most in need of a "makeover"?

__career   __income   __physical/emotional health

__day-to-day work   __living situation   __relationships, family

__education   __personal interests __relationships, platonic

__housing   __physical appearance __relationships, romantic

other: _____   _____

_____   _____

7. How important is it for you to make changes or improve on any of these areas in your life?

_____

_____

_____

_____

_____

8. What will your life be like if you aren't able to make necessary changes?

_____

_____

_____

_____

_____

9. What do you most need in order to bring about change in your life?

_____

_____

_____

_____

_____

THINGS TO THINK ABOUT

- Are the changes you want realistic, given the circumstances of your life?
- Do you have the necessary resources in your life to bring about changes you'd like to make? If not, how can you develop such resources?
- Who else might be affected by any changes you might make? In what ways?

12

Destination:
INTIMATE RELATIONSHIPS

HELEN

I just wasn't as interested in sex as I used to be. I was happy with my husband, but inside I wondered if he was still satisfied with sex. I was afraid to tell him how I felt, or ask him what he was thinking. I finally got up the nerve to talk to my doctor and learned that it wasn't all in my head. I found out that sexual arousal slows down as hormone levels drop, and that tissue in my vagina and labia is also affected by hormonal change. I was relieved to find out that she could prescribe medications to help with the physical changes. But that didn't really help with the other issues. I just didn't feel as attractive, and couldn't help but compare myself with all those other sexy and younger women I saw out there. It took me a while to realize that these issues were in my head. I finally talked to Frank, who was really supportive. After that I managed to get beyond my own self-doubts and brain washing, and found that our relationship and sex were just as good as ever. Maybe better.

IT'S IMPOSSIBLE TO talk seriously about identity and personal development without discussing relationships. In many ways, we

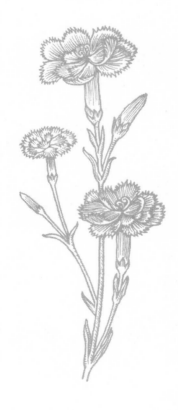

define ourselves by our relationships. How you see yourself is quite likely affected deeply by your relationships—the more positive, gratifying, and supportive relationships you've had, the more likely you are to feel good about yourself. This isn't to say that good relationships are the be-all and end-all to self-image, but they're certainly a powerful start. Although relationships were generally discussed in Chapter 11, this chapter focuses on those relationships that are of an intimate nature.

Intimacy

The meaning of intimacy varies from relationship to relationship, and even within established relationships the meaning and experience of intimacy changes over time.

Not every relationship is an intimate one. Although it can be argued that intimacy is a basic ingredient in any meaningful relationship, it's also true that there is no standard for intimacy. In fact, the meaning of intimacy varies from relationship to relationship, and even within established relationships the meaning and experience of intimacy changes over time. Not every intimate relationship is of a romantic or sexual nature. Parent-child relationships and friendships are examples of intimate relationships that are strictly platonic. In general, then, intimacy is linked more with feelings of closeness, trust, and shared experiences than with romance or sex.

However, in long-term romantic relationships, there is usually the assumption that intimacy is, or will be, linked with sexual relations. In some romantic relationships, intimacy is intertwined with and inseparable from sex. In others, intimacy is built on and reflected in shared moments and the history of the couple, and has little or nothing to do with sex. Again, there is no standard for intimacy, and no set definition of what a relationship should consist of. Intimacy is defined and experienced by the partners in a relationship, who either feel a sense of intimacy or don't. In all healthy relationships, though, romantic or platonic, intimacy is a

source of great nourishment. Take a few minutes to think about
what intimacy means to you.

INTIMATE RELATIONSHIPS

1. What does intimacy mean to you?

_____

_____

_____

_____

_____

_____

2. What are the important elements in an intimate relationship?

_____

_____

_____

_____

_____

3. In a romantic relationship, what is the difference between intimacy and sex? Is there
a difference?

_____

_____

_____

_____

_____

_____

4. Do you have intimacy in your nonsexual relationships?

_____

_____

_____

_____

5. Are you satisfied with the level of intimacy in your relationships, whether sexual or platonic?

_____

_____

_____

_____

THINGS TO THINK ABOUT

- Are you "nourished" by intimacy in your relationships or "starved" by lack of intimacy?
- If married or in a serious relationship, have you talked to your partner about intimacy? What does intimacy mean to him or her? If you haven't discussed intimacy with your partner, why not?

Importance and Meaning in Relationships

Many people find that significant relationships aren't always satisfying. A relationship with a parent or a friend, for instance, may be important in some respects but nevertheless fail to satisfy you on an emotional level. Although relationships that satisfy often become important relationships if they endure, sometimes they're short-lived or don't occupy an important place in your life. For instance, a work friendship may prove satisfying but is nonetheless unimportant in your life as a whole. The ideal personal relationship is probably one that is both important and satisfying.

As you think about intimacy in your relationships, consider your current relationships, and think about which ones are *important* and which are *satisfying*.

CURRENT RELATIONSHIPS

1. List four *important* relationships, and briefly describe why they're important:

Important Relationship	**Important Because . . .**
a. _____	_____
	_____
	_____
	_____
b. _____	_____
	_____
	_____
	_____
	_____
c. _____	_____
	_____
	_____
	_____
	_____
d. _____	_____
	_____
	_____
	_____
	_____

2. List four current relationships that are *satisfying*, and briefly describe why.

Satisfying Relationship   **What Makes This Relationship Satisfying**

a. _____   _____

                                 _____

                                 _____

                                 _____

b. _____   _____

                                 _____

                                 _____

                                 _____

                                 _____

                                 _____

c. _____   _____

                                 _____

                                 _____

                                 _____

d. _____   _____

                                 _____

                                 _____

                                 _____

                                 _____

3. List four current relationships that are dissatisfying, and briefly describe why.

Dissatisfying Relationship   **What Makes This Relationship Dissatisfying**

a. _____   _____

                                 _____

                                 _____

Dissatisfying Relationship	What Makes This Relationship Dissatisfying
b. _____	_____
	_____
	_____
	_____
c. _____	_____
	_____
	_____
	_____
d. _____	_____
	_____
	_____
	_____

4. In general, what do you seek from relationships? What makes a relationship satisfying to you?

_____

_____

_____

_____

5. What is it about a relationship that eventually makes it dissatisfying for you?

_____

_____

_____

_____

_____

6. What do you most want to change about any of your relationships in general?

_____

_____

_____

_____

THINGS TO THINK ABOUT

- Are you generally satisfied by the relationships in your life at this time? If you're not, is it easy to be honest with yourself about relationships that dissatisfy you?
- Are there some relationships in your life that may not satisfy you but are nevertheless important or permanent relationships? If so, is there anything you can do to improve the quality of these so they meet more of your needs?

Relationship Dynamics

Relational problems are often fueled by unspoken issues that can include jealousy, mistrust, unfulfilled desires, and insecurities.

The "dynamics" of a relationship—the interplay between the people in the relationship—are often unnoticed and unconscious. The underlying current of a relationship can be built on positive factors—such as love, concern, compassion, and mutual attraction. But relational problems are often fueled by unspoken issues that can include jealousy, mistrust, unfulfilled desires, and insecurities. One way to better understand relationships is to make visible otherwise hidden dynamics. This requires that you understand and see those things about your relationships that normally lie hidden under the surface but that nevertheless have an impact on (and even control over) the way the relationship goes.

As you explore your relationships, you'll be more easily able to identify what you need, what you want, and how you feel, but it will also be important to try and understand the point of view, feelings, and needs of the other person in the relationship. Relationships are a two-way street; they are not just about how you feel or what you want. The next journal entry will allow you the opportunity to explore your relationships and the sort of changes that have taken place as you've neared and entered perimenopause and midlife.

EVOLVING RELATIONSHIPS

1. Complete these sentences.

a. *My relationships have most changed because . . .* _____

_____

_____

_____

_____

_____

_____

b. *My entry into midlife has most affected my relationships because . . .* _____

_____

_____

_____

_____

_____

_____

c. *The relationships that have been affected the most are . . .* _____

_____

_____

_____

_____

_____

2. Some relationships may have been strengthened in recent years, and others in some way weakened. Think about your relationships, and why they've changed.

Strengthened Relationship   **Changed in What Way?**

_____   _____

_____   _____

_____   _____

_____   _____

_____   _____

Weakened Relationship   **Changed in What Way?**

_____   _____

_____   _____

_____   _____

_____   _____

3. Pick one of these relationships, and describe it further.

_____

4. Complete these sentences.

a. *This relationship has changed because* . . . _____

_____

_____

_____

b. *The impact of midlife changes on this relationship has been* . . . _____

_____

_____

_____

c. What I want most from this relationship is . . . _____

_____

_____

_____

_____

THINGS TO THINK ABOUT

- Do you have the power to bring about change in this relationship now? If so, how can you do this? If not, what is impeding change?
- How much energy do you put into this and other relationships? Should you put more of yourself into your relationships?

Sexuality in Relationships

We live in a relationship-oriented culture. Perhaps more to the point, we have a sex-oriented culture. It's virtually impossible to read a magazine, watch a TV situation comedy or drama, or listen to radio station without being exposed to sexual material. In the media, sexuality is often portrayed as the key element in attractiveness and relationships. Sexual taboos and boundaries have changed considerably and the sexual debate is ever present from discussions about teen parenting, safe sex, and treatment for male impotence to sexual orientation and preference.

Sex is an important factor in many relationships and an important feature in midlife change. Although some of the physical changes brought about by menopause, such as a dry vagina or loss of sexual drive, can create sexual difficulties, for the most part these are issues that are often easily overcome. Sometimes menopause actually liberates sexuality, freeing it, for example from the risk of unwanted pregnancy. And, if you have grown children, it can also mean freedom from interruptions.

Nevertheless, there are many factors that can make sex in es-

Sex is an important factor in many relationships and an important feature in midlife change.

tablished midlife relationships a difficult subject. Some of these may be the result of sexual attitudes, expectations, and practices that have developed in the relationship in the years prior to menopause. For instance, as a relationship continues to evolve during and beyond midlife, one person may want a return to sex as it was before the kids came along, and the other may not. It may be difficult to simply break away from habits formed over the course of many years. These differences become part of the issues faced by any couple in a relationship that changes over time. Discussion between partners is often the best way to begin to sort out and resolve these potential problems.

Sex and the Single Woman in Midlife

Postmenopausal women may be single for several reasons. Divorce and separation are common midlife events in our society, and it's not unusual for middle-age women to be widowed. There are also many women in midlife who have never been married. Whatever the reason, singleness, menopause, and midlife combine to create a new scenario for women who may be actively seeking or feel a need to be with a partner.

Paula Doress-Worters and Diana Siegal explore the myths of sexuality and aging in their book, *The New Ourselves, Growing Older.* It is not true that older people aren't interested in sex and no longer engage in sexual activities, that changes in hormonal levels during and after menopause inevitably cause uncomfortable sex, that women beyond their childbearing years completely lose their sexual desire, that middle-age women and beyond aren't attractive or sexually desirable, that a woman must have a male partner to have a full and complete sex life, or that the only truly satisfying sex is intercourse and vaginal orgasm. Use the next journal entry to think about sexuality in your life and in your relationship(s).

SEXUAL NEEDS

I. Answer each of the questions below, either by checking off the most appropriate answers or giving a brief answer, where asked.

SEXUAL SATISFACTION (CHECK ONE)

__satisfied with your sex life

__partly satisfied with your sex life

__mostly dissatisfied with your sex life

__dissatisfied with your sex life

RELATIONSHIP STANDING (CHECK ONE)

__in a satisfying marriage or long-term relationship

__in an unsatisfying marriage or long-term relationship

__on your own and liking it

__on your own and not liking it

PERSONAL SEXUALITY

a. Was sexuality important in the past? _____

b. How important is sexuality now?_____

c. Given other forms of sex, how important is intercourse?_____

d. How important are other forms of sexuality and intimacy, from holding hands and cuddling to manual stimulation and oral sex? _____

SEXUAL ORIENTATION

a. Has your sexual orientation changed? _____

b. If so, are you questioning why? _____

c. If so, how are you feeling about the change? _____

d. If you wish to change your orientation, can you? _____

RELATIONSHIP COMMITMENT (CHECK ALL THAT APPLY)

___If in a relationship, are you content with your partner?

___Do you want a new partner?

___Do you want an extramarital/extrarelationship partner?

___Would you rather have no partner at all?

2. Look back at the answers you've just given. What do these answers say about your sexual needs, interests, or relationships?

_____

_____

_____

_____

_____

_____

_____

_____

_____

3. What have you learned about yourself from this inventory?

_____

_____

_____

_____

_____

_____

_____

_____

_____

_____

_____

Checkpoint: Changing Relationships

Throughout this chapter, you've been thinking about your most intimate relationships and how they've changed or may be changing since your entry into midlife. In some cases, you may be feeling *proactive*: you're ready to actively change existing relationships, or even end them if they no longer fit your needs. You may even be thinking about pursuing new relationships. On the other hand, relationships may be scary for you, and you may feel like you're constantly unable to get your needs met. You may feel like you're on the "wrong" end of relationships, that you're not getting enough out of the ones you have and aren't capable of forming new relationships. If sex is involved, the situation may be even more anxiety provoking if you feel you have to perform or compete in the larger sexual market against a lot of younger women.

The next journal entry will help you take stock of your relationship needs.

You may be feeling proactive: you're ready to actively change existing relationships, or even end them if they no longer fit your needs.

CHECKPOINT: RELATIONSHIPS

1. What have you learned about your relationships?

_____

_____

_____

_____

2. What have you learned about your relationship needs?

_____

_____

_____

_____

_____

3. Do you feel in control of your relationships, or do they control you?

_____

_____

_____

_____

4. Do your relationships meet your needs for intimacy?

_____

_____

_____

_____

5. Do you feel a need to make any substantial changes in your relationships? If so, are you ready to bring about change?

_____

_____

_____

_____

_____

6. How do *you* most need to change in your relationships?

_____

_____

_____

_____

_____

THINGS TO THINK ABOUT

- Do you understand more about your relationships and your relationship needs?
- Are there some changes you need to make in your relationships? If so, can you make these changes *before* making changes in yourself?
- If you're having any significant difficulties with your intimate relationships, should you consider seeking professional help to address the situation?

13

Destination:

UNFINISHED BUSINESS

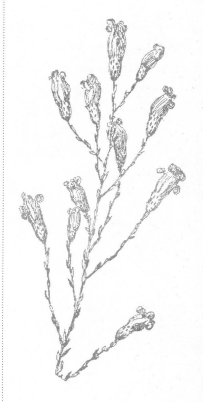

"Their errors have been weighed and found to have been dust in the balance."
—PERCY BYSSHE SHELLEY

CYNTHIA

Although I knew myself pretty well, I found myself procrastinating. I didn't know why, and it wasn't my usual way of doing things. I was intentionally putting off breast exams, doctor's visits, and even dental checkups. I figured there must be something I didn't want to find out. But since I'm pretty healthy, this didn't make sense to me. Did I unconsciously think I was sick? Did I think I had a terrible disease? Then, one night I dreamt I was dying. When I woke up I thought more about this, and found myself thinking about the dream all day. I talked to my sister that evening, and she reminded me of Janice, a mutual friend who had died eight years ago, right after she turned fifty. I was turning fifty next month! I think my mind had linked these two events and I realized her early death frightened me more than I let myself know. After this epiphany, my procrastination seemed to become a thing of the past.

GWEN

Nowadays I find myself thinking a lot about the past and things that happened to me. The death of my mother way before I was ready, my divorce and other relationships that went wrong, and how poorly I've been treated at times in my life. I think most of all of my miscarriage, and wonder what my life might have been like as a mother. I have a list of all those things that didn't go right, which just sort of piled up inside of me over the years, although I didn't realize it when it was happening. As I came into menopause, I found myself thinking more and more about how unfair my life has been and decided to talk things over with a counselor. I didn't go to many sessions, because it didn't take too long for me to realize that I had to let go of these old things and focus on the new things in my life. That wasn't such an easy thing to do, but realizing it was the first step.

To live more completely in the present and move into the future, it's important to close open books. This means finding a way to put closure on these incidents, events, and relationships and come to terms with a moment that's passed.

SOMETIMES THINKING ABOUT your future requires thinking about your past. And sometimes stepping forward into the future means putting the past away.

Many of us have powerful memories of our past, some pleasant and some not so pleasant. If you've worked sequentially through this book, you've explored some of these memories and past experiences in earlier chapters. But some past experiences may not yet be resolved; they are more like open books (or wounds). In some instances, these past experiences aren't simply memories gone by but rather are ideas that still *actively* affect and influence your behaviors, your moods, your relationships, and your life in general. Such experiences may include a relationship left incomplete or an angry feeling never fully addressed. It may be a traumatic event buried somewhere beneath your immediate consciousness or an incident you'd just rather not remember. Perhaps it's an unfulfilled relationship, a lost job, a pregnancy loss or the inability to carry a child, words never spoken to a friend who passed away, or guilt or shame about a behavior you never honestly dealt with. Whatever the scenario, this is unfinished business.

To live more completely in the present and move into the future, it's important to close open books. This means finding a way to put closure on these incidents, events, and relationships and come to terms with a moment that's passed.

Incompletion

Most people seek closure on the things in their life. If you briefly show someone a partial circle, with a small chunk missing, she or he may see it as a complete circle. The mind, seeking completion, sometimes fills in the part that's missing. Where there are holes—things missing—people strive to fill in the gap, sometimes in ways that are unhealthy and ineffective. The same is true for the unfinished business in our life.

For those unable to resolve their unfinished business, life can become an endless struggle to deal with difficult feelings. People can become emotionally stuck, unable to learn from the experience, build new relationships, and effectively move on with their lives. Often the person, situation, or thing connected to the unfinished business is no longer around or available. The moment is passed, the situation changed, the person gone. There is no one to resolve issues with—except yourself. This task of resolution is one that you'll have to work on and complete on your own. You must learn to wrap up loose ends and find a way to put closure on the situation.

Menopause and Unfinished Business

Sometimes a normal developmental time in life may act as a catalyst for old feelings and thoughts. With the transitions that come with perimenopause and menopause, it's not unusual for thoughts to return to earlier events in your life that may have evoked feelings similar to those you're experiencing now. Some of these feelings may be the stirrings of old memories, never quite forgotten and never really resolved. For some women, old feelings may re-emerge in ways that are disturbing. Even if you think you've worked out a past issue, it may return in a new form with a different intensity.

Speaking about Unfinished Business

How do you find resolution to an unresolvable situation? How do you undo something that has been irreversibly done? Part of the solution is in how you define the problem. The tasks in completing unfinished business are the tasks of self-expression, self-understanding, contemplation, and letting go. These are personal tasks. When you complete them, you will have changed nothing in the world around you, and you will have changed no one else. As you resolve unfinished business, you change yourself. Resolution is a state of mind, a perspective in which you're able to accept that which is unchangeable and through which you're able to express feelings.

The tasks in completing unfinished business are the tasks of self-expression, self-understanding, contemplation, and letting go.

Finding ways to accept and relieve yourself of feelings has much to do with giving them a voice. By "speaking" your feelings, you relieve them of the power to eat away at you. Finding a way to let go of thoughts and feelings that may otherwise remain penned up in you means finding a way to relinquish self-control, because self-expression sometimes means letting go. Sometimes it's useful to work with a therapist when letting go, but often your journal can provide that private place where you "say" the things you might not say aloud to someone else. When you voice your thoughts aloud to yourself, you are beginning the process of resolving issues with yourself. As difficult as it may be to speak out, your journal provides a private place in which you can work at your own pace, in your own time, and in your own way. Keep in mind that you're really voicing your thoughts aloud to yourself, the person you're resolving things with is *you*.

Use the next entry to think about the type of unfinished business in your life. At this point, focus only on the broad issues you may have. Don't worry about the details. Try to look at your own thoughts and get in touch with your feelings without focusing too deeply on the content and details of those thoughts or feelings.

OPEN BOOKS

1. Is the kind of closure you need more like saying good-bye to something, someone, or some time in your life, or is it more like trying to vent deep feelings that have been left unresolved?

_____

_____

_____

_____

2. What kind of unfinished business do you have? Check off all areas that apply, and add others below.

__unexpressed thoughts   __unspoken words

__unresolved feelings   __unstated regrets

__unshared experiences   __untold secrets

other: _____   _____

_____   _____

3. Of the items you checked off, think about which are about you—your thoughts and feelings, your actions, or your words—and which are about someone else—his or her feelings, actions, or words. Then complete these sentences.

a. _Unfinished business about my actions, feelings, words, or thoughts includes_ . . .

_____

_____

_____

_____

b. *Unfinished business about the actions, feelings, or words of someone else includes . . .*

_____

_____

_____

_____

4. Are your main issues about things *done* —things that you or someone did or said but perhaps shouldn't have? Or are they about things that were *never* done or said but perhaps should've been?

_____

_____

_____

_____

5. Tying up loose ends can be difficult and painful. What part will be the hardest for you?

_____

_____

_____

6. What most concerns you as you think about resolving unfinished business?

_____

_____

_____

_____

7. Do you need to complete unfinished business? If so, why?

_____

_____

_____

_____

Raising Your Voice

In the previous journal entry, you began to think about things connected to your past that are still bothering you. Thinking and writing about these things is one route you have available for getting the stuff that's inside you outside, where you can begin to deal with it. You may have a wide range of feelings and unfinished business that needs to be explored and voiced. The next journal entry is designed to help you express your feelings about your unfinished business.

FINDING YOUR VOICE

1. Describe one relationship, situation, or event that has been left open for you and that you consider unfinished business.

_____

_____

_____

_____

_____

2. When you think about this relationship or situation, how do you *feel?* Complete the sentences for each feeling that applies for you. Add other feelings you may be having, and supply explanations for all. *I feel . . .*

angry because . . . _____

apologetic because . . . _____

ashamed because . . . _____

betrayed because . . . _____

cheated because . . . _____

crushed because . . . _____

curious because . . . _____

doubtful because . . . _____

enraged because . . . _____

exploited because . . . _____

guilty because . . . _____

hurt because . . . _____

irritated because . . . _____

mistreated because . . . _____

offended because . . . _____

regretful because . . . _____

resentful because . . . _____

vengeful because . . . _____

_____ *because. . .* _____

_____ *because. . .* _____

_____ *because. . .* _____

_____ *because. . .* _____

_____ *because. . .* _____

3. Take any one of these feelings or issues, and elaborate on it. Which of these issues is most pressing for you right now?

_____

a. What makes this unfinished business for you?

_____

_____

_____

_____

_____

_____

b. What about this issue is left undone?

_____

_____

_____

_____

_____

_____

c. If this situation involves another person, what do you want to say to him or her about this piece of unfinished business?

_____

_____

_____

_____

_____

_____

_____

Expressing Regret

Addressing unfinished business doesn't necessarily require endless hours of soul-searching to find ways to resolve complex emotional issues.

Addressing unfinished business doesn't necessarily require endless hours of soul-searching to find ways to resolve complex emotional issues. Sometimes, it requires no more than voicing regret for things done or things left undone. Expressing regret isn't intended as a way to dwell on and wish away that which has passed. Instead, quite simply, it's a way to express sorrow, and sometimes remorse, for missed opportunity, a way to exorcise and relieve yourself of an otherwise unspoken burden. Expressing regret about things done or undone isn't the same as changing those things, and dealing with unresolved feelings and unsettled issues isn't about changing what was. What you are doing is changing—relieving yourself of the sometimes tremendous burden of unspoken regrets. The power of words lies in their ability to transform shapeless feelings into meaningful ideas and to bring them out into the world where they can be clearly seen.

I WISH . . .

"Thought itself needs words. It runs on them like a long wire. And if it loses the habit of words, little by little it becomes shapeless, somber."
—UGO BETTI

Complete these sentences.

1. *I wish I'd said . . .* _____

_____

2. *I wish you'd said . . .* _____

_____

3. *I wish I had . . .* _____

_____

4. *I wish I hadn't . . .* _____

_____

5. *I wish you had . . .* _____

_____

6. *I wish you hadn't . . .* _____

_____

7. *I wish I could change . . .* _____

_____

8. *I'm sorry for . . .* _____

_____

9. *I wish . . .* _____

_____

_____

10. *I wish . . .* _____

_____

_____

11. *I wish . . .* _____

_____

_____

Moving On

As you move into the final stage of your journey, you may be carrying many unresolved issues with you. It's not that you must resolve every issue and put all feelings behind you, but your ability to accept the past and the many unresolved issues and feelings that go with it is key to your ability to move into your future in a way that is emotionally healthy and unfettered by the ghosts of things gone by.

Use the final journal entry in this chapter to explore issues still to be addressed, resolve unfinished business, and otherwise let things go.

CHECKPOINT: UNFINISHED BUSINESS

1. Complete these sentences.

a. *When I look back on things unfinished, I . . .* _____

_____

_____

_____

b. *These things continue to affect me because* . . . _____

_____

_____

_____

c. *When I think of things left undone, I* . . . _____

_____

_____

_____

d. *From things left undone, I've learned* . . . _____

_____

_____

_____

2. Do you have unfinished business in your life today? Any relationships or situations that if left unattended will become the unfinished business of tomorrow?

_____

_____

_____

_____

_____

_____

_____

THINGS TO THINK ABOUT

- Are you ready to let go of old business? Do you want to let go?
- What might happen if you're unable to resolve and let go of unfinished business? Why is it so difficult to let go of the past?
- Do you need to pay attention to today's business and today's relationships?

14

Destination:

WHO WILL YOU BE?

LINDSEY

When I was younger, I couldn't imagine being "middle aged." My parents seemed so much older to me. When I was young, fifty seemed so old. Now I'm approaching that age. But I don't feel old at all. In fact, inside I feel the same as I did when I was younger—but a little wiser, a little more experienced, and a little more comfortable with myself. And that's what's so great. Even in my late forties, I still haven't "matured" to the point where I've stopped growing or know exactly who I am or want to be. I never thought of middle age as just the start, but it seems to be.

ELAINE

I felt so much energy I didn't know what to do with myself at times. With the children gone, I just dove into a frenzy of activity. At first it had a haphazard quality, and I discovered that the freedom to be something new didn't mean I knew what I wanted to be. After a while, I started the search for what had meaning for me now. It took time and energy, but it was worth it.

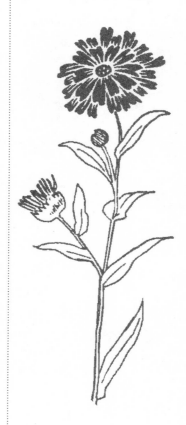

THE 1997 SURVEY of the North American Menopause Society (NAMS) reported that 52 percent of American women between the ages of forty-five and sixty view menopause as the beginning of a new and fulfilling stage of their lives, and 79 percent of peri-menopausal and postmenopausal women said they would advise other women to approach menopause with a positive attitude. The 1998 survey showed that 51 percent of American women between ages fifty and sixty-five who had reached menopause said they are happiest and most fulfilled now, as compared to when they were in their twenties, thirties, and forties. The women surveyed reported improvement in many areas of their lives since menopause, including family and home life, personal fulfillment, focus on hobbies and other interests, relationships with their spouse or partner, and friendships. Approximately three-quarters of women also reported making some type of lifestyle change at middle age or menopause, including changes in diet or nutritional habits, exercise, and reducing their stress level. The executive director of NAMS reported, "When we ask women, we continually hear that they view menopause as the beginning of many positive changes in their lives and health."

By now you're in the final stages of your journey through menopause. In this journal, you've had the opportunity to think about menopause and the role it has and will play in your life and in shaping your future. You've written about a variety of ways in which you see and understand yourself and others, and you've considered medical, health, and other interventions and whether they fit your particular situation, lifestyle, or value system.

Of course, this is one journey that doesn't really have a final destination. Menopause is a passage from one part of your life to the next, and this journey "ends" only when you feel ready to move into the second half of your life where the rest of your journey begins. In this chapter, you'll have the chance to think about what's ahead on your journey. Of this journey, the Bengali

Approximately three-quarters of women . . . reported making some type of lifestyle change at middle age or menopause, including changes in diet or nutritional habits, exercise, and reducing their stress level.

poet, writer, and composer Rabindranath Tagore said, "When we rejoice in our fullness, then we can part with our fruits with joy."

Decisions and Choices

Some things *never* change. Your life is always going to be full of decisions and choices. In some ways, decision making about your life can be summed up this simply: as your life is changing or has already changed, where do you want to be, what do you want to be doing, and who do you want to be doing it with? No doubt, you face and are limited by many real-life constraints—parenting, work, relationships, finances, and other things over which you don't necessarily have full control. These make up the backdrop of your life against which decisions are made. Within that context, there's usually no way to advise you of the "correct" decision or the "right" course to take. In fact, there's often more than one "correct" decision and more than one "wrong" choice. But there are guidelines to decision making that can help you to think about and arrive at an *appropriate* decision.

Some decisions are not really choices at all but rather requirements, especially when attached to personal responsibility.

As you think about your choices and appropriate decisions, consider that many of them have consequences, certainly to yourself and possibly to others. When making decisions and choices, keep in mind three factors:

1. *Responsibility.* Some decisions are not really choices at all but rather are requirements, especially when attached to personal responsibility. If you're a parent, for instance, you have decisions that must be made to ensure the health and safety of your children. But even required decisions are avoidable to those willing to deny their responsibilities. As you plan for and move forward into your future, consider who will be affected by your decisions and for whom you may be responsible.

2. *Spontaneity versus impetuousness.* Sometimes there's no reason in the world to not act on a whim or make a quick choice. It's healthy to be spontaneous at times. However, sometimes acting without thinking can be impetuous and foolhardy. Where spontaneity is generally thought of as harmless and even refreshing, we usually think of impetuous behavior as thoughtless and potentially problematic. As you make decisions, think about the difference between being spontaneous and being impetuous. Decisions that affect your life and the lives of others need to be carefully considered.

3. *Long-term effects.* Finally, take into account that decisions you make now may have effects that stay with you a long time. Buying a new wardrobe of clothes, seeking a new career, or moving from one home to another in the same community may involve some deep decision making, but none necessarily represents a radical change. On the other hand, selling your home and moving to another state, leaving your husband or partner, or giving up your job are far more significant decisions in terms of their long-term impact and are often difficult decisions to later reverse.

Use the next journal entry to explore your approach to decision making.

DECISIONS AND CHOICES

1. Think about current decisions and choices in your life. What sort of decisions are the hardest to make?

_____

_____

_____

_____

2. In what ways has menopause or midlife led to the sort of choices you're facing?

_____

_____

_____

3. In what ways has menopause or midlife opened up the possibility of change?

_____

_____

_____

4. What opportunities for change are in your life right now?

_____

_____

_____

5. What are the risks of change?

_____

_____

_____

_____

6. Who else will be affected by your decisions, and in what ways?

_____

_____

_____

THINGS TO THINK ABOUT

- Are you afraid of change or excited by it? Do your fears about change outweigh the opportunities?
- Are you at a point in your life where you can spot opportunity for change? What can you do to increase your ability to see such opportunities?

Moving Forward

What sort of choices are you facing now as you move forward, and what sort of decisions are you making? Are you opting to stay the same, or are you considering major changes in your life or relationships? Is moving on simply a matter of a new attitude, is it a shift in the things you do, or does it involve a restructuring of your life? If you have the freedom to make decisions without regard for anyone else (such as children, spouse, or financial obligations), are you thinking about changing jobs, going back to school, traveling the world, or moving across country?

Recognize that you do have choices.

Although there is no right or wrong here, there are steps that can help you arrive at decisions that are appropriate for your lifestyle and responsibilities.

- *Recognize that you do have choices.* Much of the time, you're not simply a passive agent in a world where things have to be a certain way.

- *Consider the nature of the problem that you're trying to resolve.* Every decision is a response to a particular situation: what's the issue, problem, or situation you want to address?

- *Consider all options.* Think of every possible alternative, including the outlandish ones. In this step, your job is to be creative—what decisions might you make?

- *Evaluate your choices.* Think about those choices that you can realistically make right now. If only one choice comes up, you may even come up with a clear decision at this point.

- *Think about the consequences.* What are the cons of your decision options? Who will be affected by your choice, and how? How will your possible choices affect your life, your finances, your relationships, and so on?

- *Take time for reflection.* Think carefully about the decision you're planning to make. What will it feel like to actually take those steps and make that choice? What will it feel like to not make that choice? Is the decision you're pondering permanent, or is it reversible?

The next journal entry is intended to help you think about individual decision choices, as well as your decision-making style in general. Follow the general model for decision making described above. This is a framework you can use to think about and map out solutions for almost any issue in your life from relationship choices to decisions about changes in your lifestyle.

MAKING DECISIONS

1. Briefly describe one decision you're currently pondering.

_____

_____

_____

2. List six different choices for resolving this issue.

a. _____   d. _____

b. _____   e. _____

c. _____   f. _____

3. Review the possible choices you've just identified, and select the three most realistic choices. For each, complete these sentences to indicate how this choice could fit the circumstances and reality of your life.

a. *This solution fits because* . . . _____

_____

b. *This solution fits because* . . . _____

_____

c. *This solution fits because* . . . _____

_____

4. Select just one of these choices, and use it as the focal point for the remainder of this entry. (You might want to repeat this entry several times in order to think through each of the possible choices you identified.)

_____

5. What are possible consequences of this choice? Is there a price to pay?

_____

_____

_____

_____

6. How will your life be affected by this choice?

_____

_____

_____

_____

7. Who else's life will be affected by this decision, and how?

_____

_____

_____

_____

THINGS TO THINK ABOUT

- Do you better understand the issues and choices involved in this decision? What stops you from making a choice and acting on it in this case?
- Can you afford to take a chance on this decision, or are the consequences irreversible?
- Are you acting too quickly on decisions without giving them ample thought, or are you not acting quickly enough?

Negative Tapes

If you're not yet content with the path your life has taken or the path ahead, the chances are that you have some old "tapes" you're playing to yourself. We all have them—the negative tapes we play in our minds that often hark back to early teachings, reprimands, failures, and fears. They may be completely untrue, outdated, and a reflection of our worst fears and greatest insecurities, but they still affect our movement toward goals not yet attained. Take some time to review any possible negative tapes you may be playing, then complete the next journal entry.

The negative tapes we play in our minds often hark back to early teachings, reprimands, failures, and fears.

NEGATIVE TAPES

1. What is one negative message you tell yourself when you attempt to move forward?

_____

_____

_____

_____

2. In what ways does this message hold you back?

_____

_____

_____

_____

3. Does this message contribute to your overall stress? If so, how?

_____

_____

_____

_____

4. Do you recall where or how you learned this negative message?

_____

_____

_____

_____

_____

5. Is it logical or rational?

_____

_____

_____

_____

6. Is the negative message true?

_____

_____

_____

_____

7. How can you stop playing this tape?

_____

_____

_____

_____

_____

Looking Back as You Move Ahead

You've by now had the chance to think about and express your feelings and thoughts about this passage of life, explore life as you enter its middle years, wrap up unfinished business, and consider where you're heading. As you near the end of this journal, it's important to provide a way to wrap up this part of your journey, even as you move on into your future. For all you've said and written already, what still needs to be said? What do you want to tell others about what you've been through on your healing journey, how you're feeling now, and how it's affected you?

REFLECTIONS ON YOUR JOURNEY

*"No spring, nor summer beauty hath such grace,
As I have seen in one autumnal face."*
——JOHN DUNNE

Complete these sentences.

1. *I've most learned . . .* _____

_____

_____

_____

_____

_____

2. *My journey through menopause has taught me* . . . _____

_____

_____

_____

_____

_____

_____

_____

_____

3. *My journey through menopause has left me feeling* . . . _____

_____

_____

_____

_____

_____

_____

_____

_____

4. *The most bitter part of my journey has been . . .* _____

_____

_____

_____

_____

_____

_____

_____

_____

_____

_____

5. *The sweetest part of my journey has been . . .* _____

_____

_____

_____

_____

_____

_____

_____

_____

_____

_____

6. I most look forward to . . . _____

_____

_____

_____

_____

_____

_____

_____

_____

7. I most need to say . . . _____

_____

_____

_____

_____

_____

_____

_____

_____

THINGS TO THINK ABOUT

- Have you been able to accept this change of life and your passage into midlife?
- What has this journey most taught you about yourself and your life in general?

15

As One Journey Ends, Another Begins

IT'S DIFFICULT TO say when any journey really ends. Even though you've come to the end of this book, your journal is never really complete unless you choose never to write again. What you've been through and what you've learned through your journaling work sets the pace for the journey that's ahead. If your experience with menopause has left you wiser, stronger, and more confident than ever then you're in good shape for the things that are yet to come. If your journey has left you emotionally shaky and uncertain, consider getting outside help. You don't have to be experiencing emotional difficulties to get help dealing with unresolved issues, uncertainties, and life decisions. Individual counseling provides a useful vehicle for exploring many life issues. Support groups also offer a cooperative, communal, and sensitive environment for sharing and interacting with others in similar situations. If you have experienced physical problems or difficulties, don't hesitate to speak to your physician, nurse practitioner, or other health care provider.

Where will your life take you now? If you've consistently used your journal through your menopause, then you've hopefully

"Who wants to become a writer? And why? Because it's the answer to everything. To 'Why am I here?' To uselessness. It's the streaming reason for living. To note, to pin down, to build up, to create, to be astonished at nothing, to cherish the oddities, to let nothing go down the drain, to make something, to make a great flower out of life, even if it's a cactus."
—ENID BAGNOLD

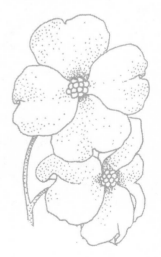

You don't have to be experiencing emotional difficulties to get help dealing with unresolved issues, uncertainties, and life decisions.

found it a useful tool that has served many purposes: a place to express or explore feelings, or both; a guide to help direct you through menopause and help shape your decisions; a narrative of your life during a major change; a mirror to reflect your relationships and interactions with others; a means of learning new ways to see yourself and the world around you. Will your journal continue to be a valuable companion as you continue along your lifelong journey? This final journal entry will help you answer this question.

MY JOURNAL

1. How has your journal been most useful?

_____

_____

_____

_____

_____

2. Have certain types of journal entries been more useful than others?

_____

_____

_____

_____

_____

3. What's been the most difficult aspect of journaling for you?

_____

_____

_____

_____

_____

4. What's been the most fulfilling aspect of journaling?

_____

_____

_____

_____

_____

5. Describe your overall experience of keeping this journal.

_____

_____

_____

_____

_____

_____

6. Complete this sentence. *My journal* . . . _____

_____

_____

_____

_____

_____

_____

_____

_____

_____

_____

_____

In completing this book you've accomplished a great deal and taken significant steps down the path to self-help and personal growth. Although your personal journey will likely never be complete, the lessons and methods learned in this book will help you along the way. If you've found the entries in this journal useful, you may want to explore other books in this series, particularly *The Healing Journey* and *The Healing Journey for Couples*. Both of these books provide more general journal-writing exercises that are focused on self-exploration and personal growth.

Where will your healing journey take you next, and what tools or people will you need to help take you along that path?

Resources

American Medical Association. *Complete Guide to Women's Health*. New York: Random House, 1996.

Apter, Terri. *Secret Paths: Women in the New Midlife*. New York: Norton, 1997.

Bonnick, Sydney. *The Osteoporosis Handbook: Every Woman's Guide to Prevention and Treatment*. Dallas, TX: Taylor, 1997.

Borton, Joan. *Drawing from the Women's Well: Reflections on the Life Passage of Menopause*. San Diego, CA: Lura Media, 1992.

Borysenko, Joan. *Minding the Body, Mending the Mind*. New York: Bantam, 1993.

Cabot, Sandra. *Smart Medicine for Menopause*. Garden City Park, NY: Avery, 1995.

Domar, Alice. *Healing Mind, Healthy Woman*. New York: Delta, 1997.

Doress-Worters, Paula, and Diana Siegal. *The New Ourselves, Growing Older*. New York: Touchstone, 1994.

Dosh, Robert. *The Taking Care of Menopause Workbook*. Oakland, CA: New Harbinger, 1997.

Goldberg, Burton. *Alternative Medicine: The Definitive Guide*. Tiburon, CA: Future Medicine Publishing Group, 1998.

Goldsworthy, Joanna. *A Certain Age: Reflecting on Menopause*. New York: Columbia University Press, 1994.

Greenwood, Sadja. *Menopause Naturally: Preparing for the Second Half of Life*. Volcano, CA: Volcano Press, 1996.

Greer, Germaine. *The Change: Woman, Aging, and the Menopause*. New York: Fawcett Columbine, 1991.

Jacobowitz, Ruth. *150 Most Asked Questions about Menopause*. New York: Hearst, 1993.

Lark, Susan. *Dr. Susan Lark's The Menopause Self-Help Book*. Berkeley, CA: Celestial Arts, 1996.

Love, Susan. *Dr. Susan Love's Hormone Book*. New York: Random House, 1998.

Lucks, Naomi, and Melene Smith. *A Woman's Midlife Companion: The Essential Resource for Every Woman's Journey*. Rocklin, CA: Prima, 1997.

Northrup, Christiane. *Women's Bodies, Women's Wisdom*. New York: Bantam, 1998.

Ojeda, Linda. *Menopause without Medicine*. Alameda, CA: Hunter House, 1995.

Reichman, Judith. *I'm Too Young to Get Old: Health Care for Women after Forty*. New York: Times Books, 1997.

Sheehy, Gail. *The Silent Passage*. New York: Pocket Books, 1998.

Teaff, Nancy Lee, and Kim Wright Wiley. *Perimenopause: Preparing for the Change*. Rocklin, CA: Prima, 1996.

Weed, Susun. *Menopausal Years: The Wise Woman Way*. Woodstock, N.Y.: Ash Tree, 1992.

Weil, Andrew. *Spontaneous Healing*. New York: Ballantine, 1996.

Williams, Mark. *The American Geriatric Society's Complete Guide to Aging and Health*. New York: Harmony Books, 1995.

Self-Help and Consumer Health Organizations

Boston Women's Health Collective
240A Elm St.
Boston, MA 02144
617-625-0271

National Women's Health Network
1325 G St. NW
Washington, DC 20005
202-347-1140

North American Menopause Society
P. O. Box 94527
Cleveland, OH 44101
216-844-8748

Women's Health Initiative Program Office
1 Rockledge Centre, Suite 300, MS 7966
6705 Rockledge Dr.
Bethesda, MD 20892-7966
301-402-2900

About the Authors

PHIL RICH, EdD, MSW, DCSW, holds a doctorate in applied behavioral and organizational studies and is a clinical social worker diplomate with a master's degree in social work. Over the past two decades, he has worked as a director of treatment programs, a clinical supervisor, and a practicing therapist in both the outpatient and inpatient setting. He currently maintains a private practice in western Massachusetts in addition to his position as a clinical director. He is the primary author and series editor of the seven books in the *Healing Journey* series.

FRANCES MERVYN, BScN, PhD, is on faculty at the Massachusetts School of Professional Psychology, where she teaches community psychology and consultation. She has been in the community health—mental health field for over three decades. Beginning as a public health nurse in Canada, she continued her education at Harvard University where she received a master's degree in education and at Boston College where she received her doctorate in psychology. She was Director at the Human Relations Service in Wellesley, the first community health center in the nation. Currently she is the Continuing Education Director at the Boston Institute for the Development of Infants and Parents, maintains an active clinical and consultation practice, and presents ongoing seminars on menopause.